A Practical Guide to Technology in Dentistry

Nicolas M. Jedynakiewicz

Lecturer in Clinical Dental Science
Academic Unit of Dental Bioengineering
University of Liverpool
England

Wolfe Publishing

Published in 1992 by Wolfe Publishing, an imprint of Mosby–Year Book Europe Ltd
Printed by BPCC Hazells Ltd , Aylesbury, England.
ISBN 0 7234 1742 X

A CIP catalogue record for this book is available from the British Library.

For full details of all Mosby–Year Book Europe Ltd titles please write to Mosby–Year Book Ltd, Brook House, 2–16 Torrington Place, London WC1E 7LT, England.

Contents

TO RYSZARD AND ELIZABETH

Foreword

The last decade has witnessed very considerable changes in the concepts and techniques of dentistry and the emergence of a paradox of intellectual and practical importance. The over-emphasis on the mechanical aspects of dentistry so apparent in undergraduate teaching ten or so years ago has given way to a biological approach in which intervention is avoided if possible or minimised if appropriate. At the same time as this trend has become apparent, it has become equally obvious that the efficacy of operative dentistry and the quality of the work performed can only be improved if the technology applied becomes more and more sophisticated. The paradox is self-evident as traditional dental technology is reduced in relevence but successful dental treatment relies increasingly on the application of new, innovative and often highly complex technology of the 1990s.

Because of the practical nature of dental treatment, the dental profession has always encompassed technical skills as well as intellectual rigour. As the trends outlined above move apace and the available technology emerges even faster, so it is necessary for the dentist and his staff to be made aware, and to maintain awareness, of the technological resources available. It has been estimated that the half-life of knowledge in some technical areas is less than three years; that is, half of what is learnt today will be wholly redundant within three years (or perhaps even shorter in some areas of information technology). It is therefore highly appropriate that a practical guide to dental technology, in all its aspects, should be published so that members of this profession can understand the state-of-the-art with their facilities.

I know of no better person to write and assemble such a book as my colleague Nicolas Jedynakiewicz. While maintaining a most healthy attitude towards the concepts and practices of preventive dentistry and minimal intervention, he has been most astute in his perceptions of when technology can be used and how it may be used most effectively, in both conventional and advanced forms of restorative dentistry. These attitudes become obvious on reading this book and I hope that it will both inspire and reassure countless readers who wish to know more about the instruments and machines that they use, or should use.

David Williams
Professor of Dental Science
Departments of Clinical Engineering and
Clinical Dental Science
University of Liverpool.

Preface

Technology in dentistry is increasing in sophistication and also in cost. The practising dentist has a need to understand how equipment works and what its limitations are. Such an understanding should lead to the clinician working in harmony with his or her technology and instruments. Equipment which is not abused should give many more years of service than it would if ill-treated. Well-maintained, high quality equipment, used correctly, helps the dentist provide a high quality of operative care.

This book is written to provide an explanation of dental equipment and a guide to its selection and use. There are few other books which deal with this subject and the scope of its contents presented me with some difficulty. Those who looked at this book in its early stages asked that it should include other technology which the dentist is likely to encounter in connection with his or her profession. This resulted in the chapters on communication, computers and photographic equipment. The scope of dentistry and dental practice is very wide, so I hope that those reading this book may let me know their ideas for future editions. Altogether, I hope that within these pages there will be information of value to dentists, hygienists, dental assistants and technicians, research workers and others.

Special thanks are due to my friend and colleague Nicolas Martin who suggested that I write this book in the first place, helped me create its outline structure and badgered me with encouragement until it was finished. Thanks are due also to Judith Fletcher and many other colleagues who helped me with advice and information. I am also grateful for the patient help from Patrick Daly on behalf of the publishers.

Nicolas M. Jedynakiewicz

CHAPTER 1

The Dental Operatory

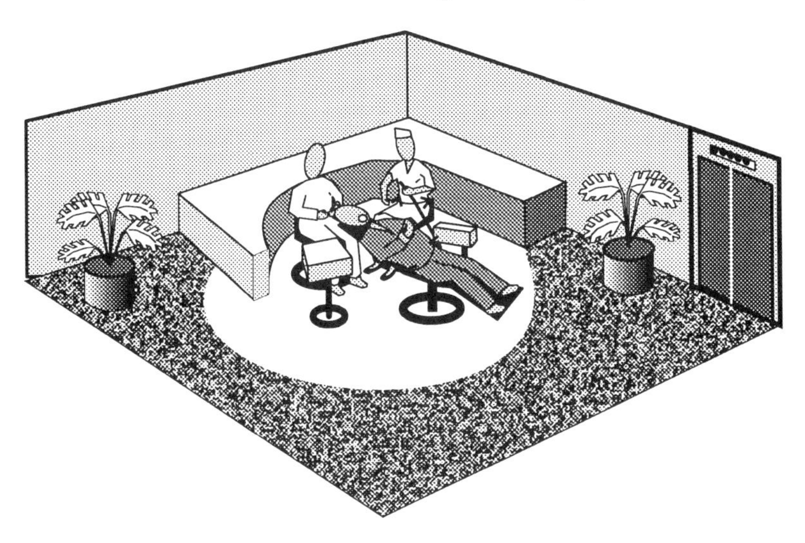

Fig. 1. The dental operatory.

A standard modern dental operatory consists of an instrument delivery unit, a dental chair with powered movements, a dental light and an assistant's unit providing suction etc. *(Fig. 1)*. Custom-designed cabinetry provides easy access work-surfaces and storage areas for the various materials and instruments which are required in the course of operative treatment. There will be in addition a number of auxiliary devices which are necessary for specific procedures and these will vary according to the particular specialty of the practitioner. Above all, the design of the surgery and the equipment must ensure comfortable and safe working conditions for the dentist and staff and facilitate efficient running of the practice.

The design of the operatory must permit effective control of cross-infection and allow ease of cleaning and disinfection. This should be the first priority in the design considerations for new and upgraded surgeries.

The materials and fabrics used in the interior design should be selected carefully for optimum performance. Surfaces should be durable and able to withstand chemical spillage without stain or damage. They should be cleaned easily without the need for expensive cleaning methods and should maintain their properties over a long life-span of regular, thorough cleaning. They should resist the build-up of contaminants and should not trap particulate matter. It may sometimes be difficult to achieve good aesthetics whilst maintaining these stringent requirements, but performance-related properties should always be placed first. The dentist would be wise to take samples of any material proposed for work-surfaces etc. and check that they do resist the range of chemicals which he may use or spill on them. Changing a whole work-surface because of one unfortunate unsightly stain can be a very expensive matter.

Services

The dental operatory requires a wide range of power and other services. Electricity, gas, compressed air and mains water must be supplied to various points. Drainage and forced vacuum systems must be installed. Additionally, telephone lines, internal intercom systems and computer data and network lines are needed. The detailed mechanism of provision of each of these services is dealt with later in this book.

The Instrument Delivery Unit

The instrument delivery unit provides powered instruments to the dentist. A minimum configuration would consist of an air turbine, a micro-motor and a triple syringe. Additional options would include further turbines or motors, an ultrasonic scaler, and electrosurgery handpiece, fibre-optic diagnostic lighting and a curing light for resin materials.

The unit supplies controlled compressed air, coolant water, fibre lighting and electricity according to the needs of the instruments on-board. It switches the supply to the instrument in use and provides control of flow by a foot pedal.

There are many designs of instrument delivery systems, all of which purport to be the most ergonomic. Overall, the system of choice is the one which best suits the operating methods and design perception of the dentist who is using it *(Fig. 2)*.

Instruments can be delivered from the side of the dental chair, from a cabinet adjacent to the chair, from a trolley next to the chair, from behind the chair or from over the top of the patient. The most popular configuration is from the side of the chair in the form of a trolley or a unit on an arm.

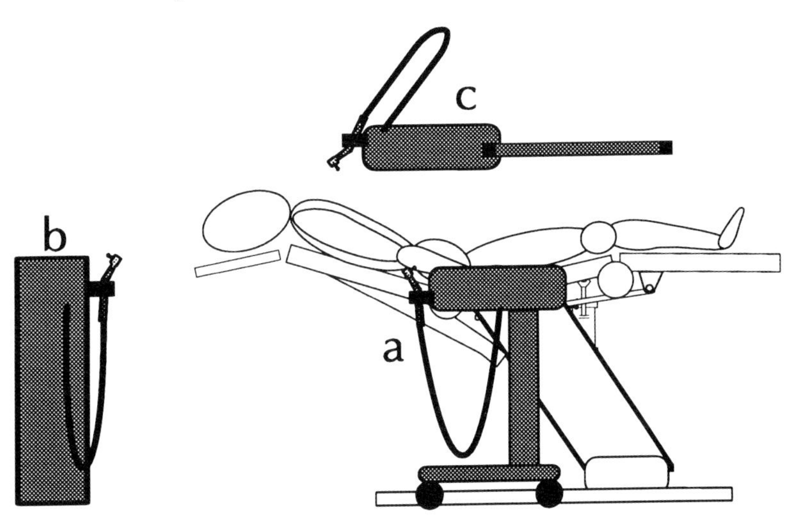

Fig. 2. Instrument delivery units: (a) side delivery; (b) rear delivery; (c) over the patient delivery.

It is imperative that the dental unit is designed to minimise cross-infection in all respects. All surfaces of the unit must be easy to clean and disinfect. Handpieces must be sterilisable and any component remaining on the unit, such as the micro-motor, must be either covered by a removable shield or must be disinfected easily.

Cooling water is supplied to the handpieces by the dental unit and this may be a major source of cross-infection. Stagnant water in the pipe-work of the unit can be a ready reservoir of micro-organisms. It is vital that an effective throughput is maintained and that back-flow from infected handpieces is resisted. One of the problems with cooling water flow is that the control valve is buried in the system unit and connected to the handpiece via a flexible and elastic hose. This hose expands slightly under the pressure of the flowing coolant and then contracts elastically when the coolant valve switches off the supply. This means that when the dentist lifts his foot off the foot control the water flow does not stop immediately. The collapse of the elastic supply tubing creates a dribble of water for some seconds after the instrument has stopped turning. To eliminate this feature, many units incorporate a 'suck-back' valve which operates for a few seconds every time the instrument is stopped. This produces a negative pressure in the water line so that it is emptied rapidly and does not dribble. The overwhelming disadvantage of this system is that it sucks in contaminated water from the handpiece and introduces infective material into the system unit. The next time the machine is activated this infected water is sprayed out. Despite the obvious hazard of such a circuit, most dental units today incorporate suck-back valves.

Some dental units incorporate a reservoir into which a mild disinfectant can be loaded. This is injected into the coolant water to help reduce the micro-organism count. However, the consequences of the dental personnel breathing such aerosols over a long period must be considered.

Aesthetics are as important as ergonomics in the selection of a dental unit. A fearsome unit hanging over the patient like the sword of Damocles is hardly a practice builder. Many dentists favour a low-level unit out of the line of sight of the patient in the chair so as to maintain a non-threatening environment.

Over the patient delivery has many ergonomic advantages. Instruments are available with minimal hand movement and can be accessed by the dental assistant as well. The assistant can change burs for the dentist and speed up work efficiency.

Features of dental units

Handpiece selection

Operation of the appropriate drive circuits for each handpiece may be selected manually or automatically when the handpiece is picked up. The most sophisticated units utilise infra-red sensors to detect when a handpiece leaves its holder. Some units allow switching out of the remaining handpieces so that while one handpiece is in use another may be picked up without being activated so that the head assembly or bur can be changed. Where the instrument delivery unit shares microcomputer control with the chair, an interlock is provided so that the chair cannot be operated and the patient moved whist the instruments are in use.

Chip-blower

A chip-blower is an extra control system in the instrument supply unit which directs a stream of air through the turbine cooling lines in order to blast away any debris left in the cavity after cutting. The cavity may be dried as well. The idea is to reduce the number of hand movements by decreasing the number of times the triple syringe is used. The chip-blower is activated by an extra foot control. The best units run a secondary line for chip air so that the air-jet is sufficiently powerful to be useful.

The dental chair

Dental chairs vary considerably in their range of movements. A minimum of height control and back-rest drop is needed for most purposes although the simplest system consists of a reclined flat chair with a height adjustment. Ideally, the chair should include height control, back-rest drop, head-rest height and tilt and trendelenberg tilt *(Figs 3 and 4)*.

It should be borne in mind that a power failure will lead to arrest of action of the dental chair. Some dental chairs designed for use in oral surgery units incorporate a manual release valve to allow the chair to be reclined into a resuscitation position without the need for power.

Whilst some dental chairs are built with a sizable base which makes the unit inherently stable, most require bolting to the floor to ensure that they do not tip over in use. It is important to ensure that the floor can stand the load and that firm anchoring points are available for bolting down.

Electrical safety in general is considered later, but it is worth emphasising at this point that the power circuit to the dental chair should be protected with a residual current circuit breaker to ensure maximum safety in operation.

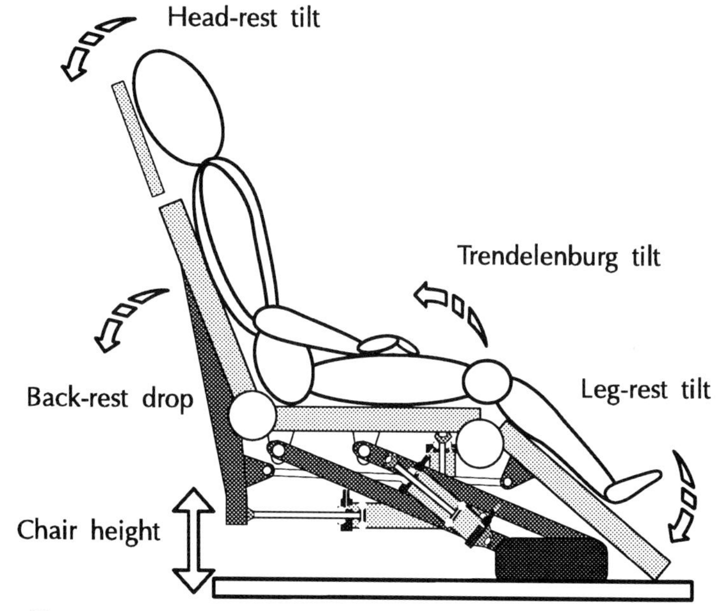

Fig. 3. Movements of a dental chair.

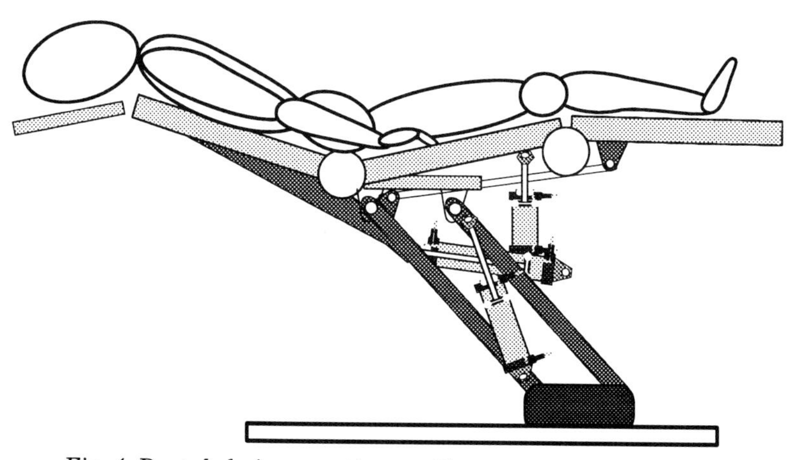

Fig. 4. Dental chair: operating position.

The hinge position of the dental chair should coincide with the hinge axis of the patient's hips. If this is not done then as the back-rest is dropped the patient gets a somewhat unpleasant feeling of being stretched in the middle.

More sophisticated models also incorporate longitudinal compensation for back-rest drop. As the back-rest of the chair is reclined, the horizontal position of the patient's head moves significantly and in a surgery which has been designed rather tightly from an ergonomic aspect, this can be unacceptable. By mounting the chair top on rails, it can be slid along over the base in order to compensate. The effect is one of the patient's head moving vertically no matter which chair movement is engaged. Complex chair movement can be used to tilt the angle of the patient's head without altering the vertical position.

Dental chairs must be capable of lifting considerable weights and therefore involve the use of powerful motors and gears. However, such power can cause great damage if misdirected so safety aspects of design must be addressed carefully.

Two methods of achieving chair movement are in common use, screw jacks and hydraulic jacks.

Screw lift

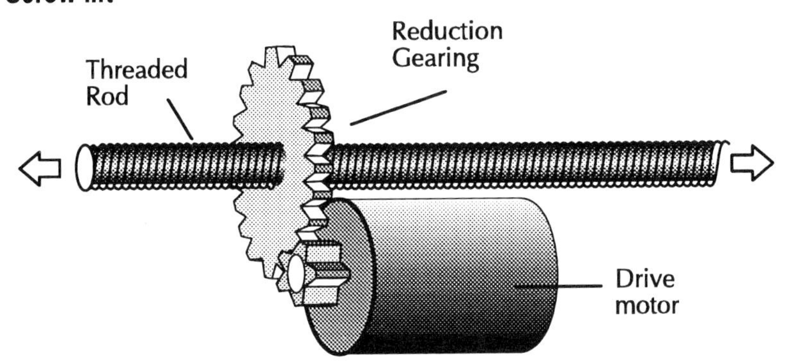

Fig. 5. Screw-driven lift mechanism.

Screw-lift mechanisms are the simplest way of operating a dental chair. They utilise a threaded shaft which rotates inside a collar to drive two chair components apart or to bring them closer together *(Figs 5 and 6)*. The screw lift is usually cheaper to manufacture than hydraulic systems except in more complex systems when the need for a motor for each movement increases the cost over the single-motor hydraulic type. With a modern refined design it offers quiet and efficient operation. By making the collar from machinable polymers, wear is minimised and the main components become maintenance free as lubrication is not needed.

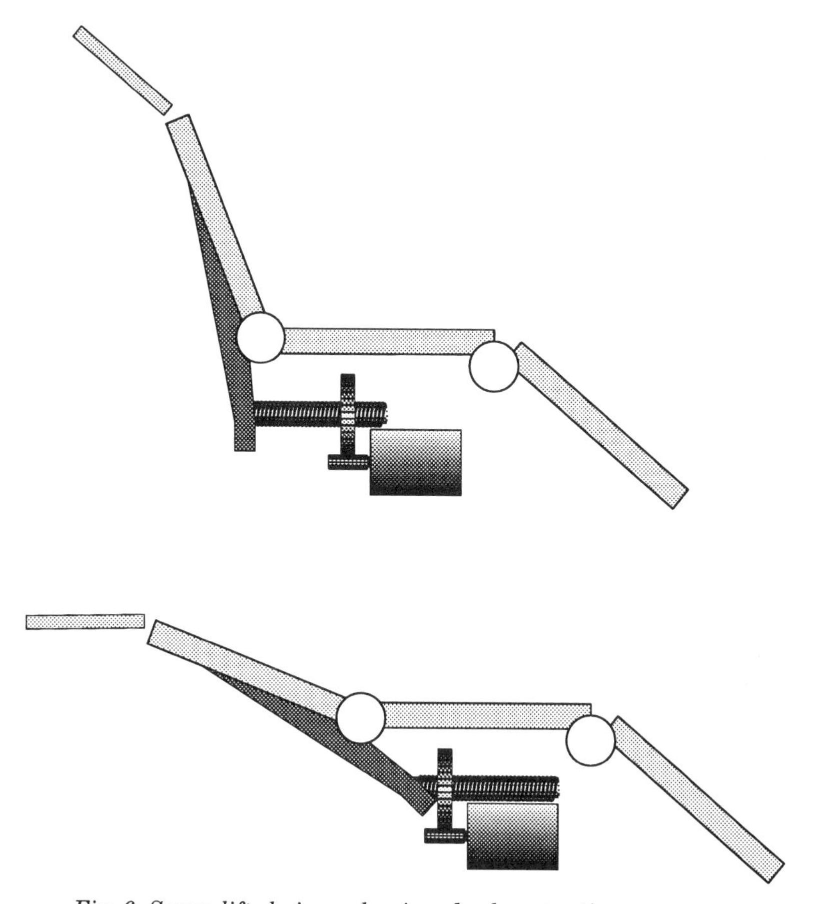

Fig. 6. Screw-lift chair mechanism; back-rest action.

Hydraulic lift

The hydraulic lift is one of the most common ways of operating a dental chair. The basic component is the hydraulic servo *(Fig. 7)*. This is powered through a system of switchable valves by an hydraulic pump. Hydraulic lifts are extremely smooth in operation and have the advantage of needing only one motor to power all the movement functions of the chair.

The hydraulic servo consists of a piston in a cylinder. Hydraulic oil can be pumped in at either end to move the piston. 'O-ring' seals allow a polished rod which is attached to the piston to move out of the cylinder. The end of this rod and the opposite end of the cylinder are mounted between the components to be moved.

An oil compressor is powered by an electric motor and recirculates hydraulic oil through the system *(Fig. 8).* Forward and reverse movement of the servo and selection of individual servos is achieved by means of valves which switch the flow of oil between the components *(see Fig. 110).* The valves are generally electrically operated so that sophisticated control systems such as chair position memory can be used.

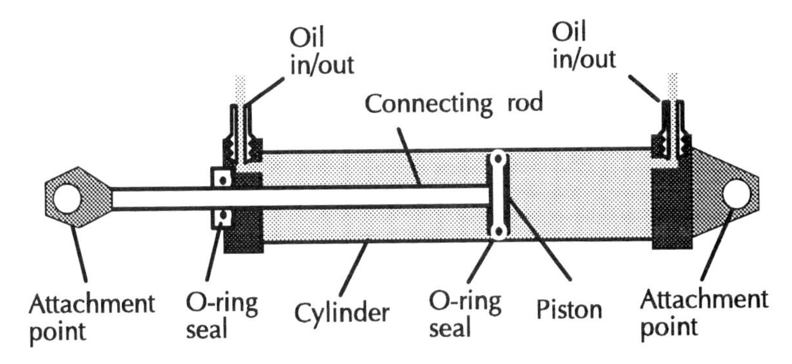

Fig. 7. Hydraulic servo.

The action of the hydraulic servo is translated into movement of the chair by means of levers. Some chairs use interlinked levers to achieve co-ordinated movements from a single servo. Such movements may be the dropping of the chair back-rest *(Fig. 9)* combined with trendelenburg tilt of the whole chair top.

Chair height control requires the most powerful servos because there is no scope for counter-balancing. The most common lifting system is the pantograph chair base *(Fig. 10).* Two lever arms support the chair top and by virtue of this geometry the top remains parallel to the floor whilst the levers lift it. The servo can be mounted diagonally across the levers to actuate the lift.

Safety considerations are paramount in the design of chair lift mechanisms. It is important that the patient cannot be raised vertically against immovable objects and that the chair cannot be lowered under power onto the dentist's or assistant's feet. Because of the potential danger of the pantograph base crushing feet it is usual to build pressure-detecting micro-switches into a pad which sits on the floor under the danger zones of the chair. Some systems lower the patient by releasing the system to the effects of gravity rather than actually powering the chair downwards. In this way the maximum force which the system can produce is the weight of the patient plus the weight of the chair top. This can still be very considerable.

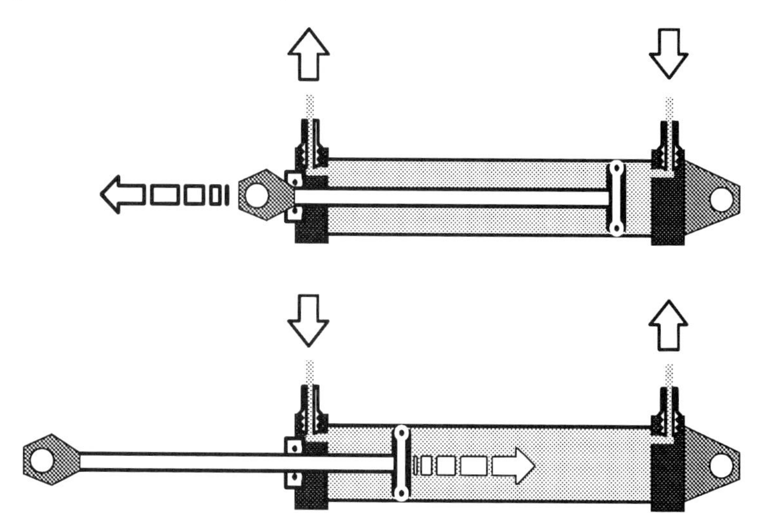

Fig. 8. Operation of the hydraulic servo; movement of oil forces the piston to move within the cylinder. A connecting arm links the piston to the component to be moved.

A sophisticated feature of some dental units is the electronic interlocking of the handpiece controls with those of the dental chair mechanism. This prevents the chair mechanism from being activated if any handpiece is in use. This useful safety feature should be far more prevalent in the design of dental units than it is.

Programmed action

Many dental chairs incorporate a circuit which allows one or more positions of the dental chair to be recorded in a memory and then selected at the touch of a button. The simplest system use switches incorporated into the chair base which trip when the chair reaches a preset position. The position of the switches, and hence the preselected position of the chair, is set by the engineer who installs the unit and cannot be changed easily. The most sophisticated control system records the information electronically in a microcomputer memory and can be altered easily by the clinician. Several positions can be recorded in the better chairs.

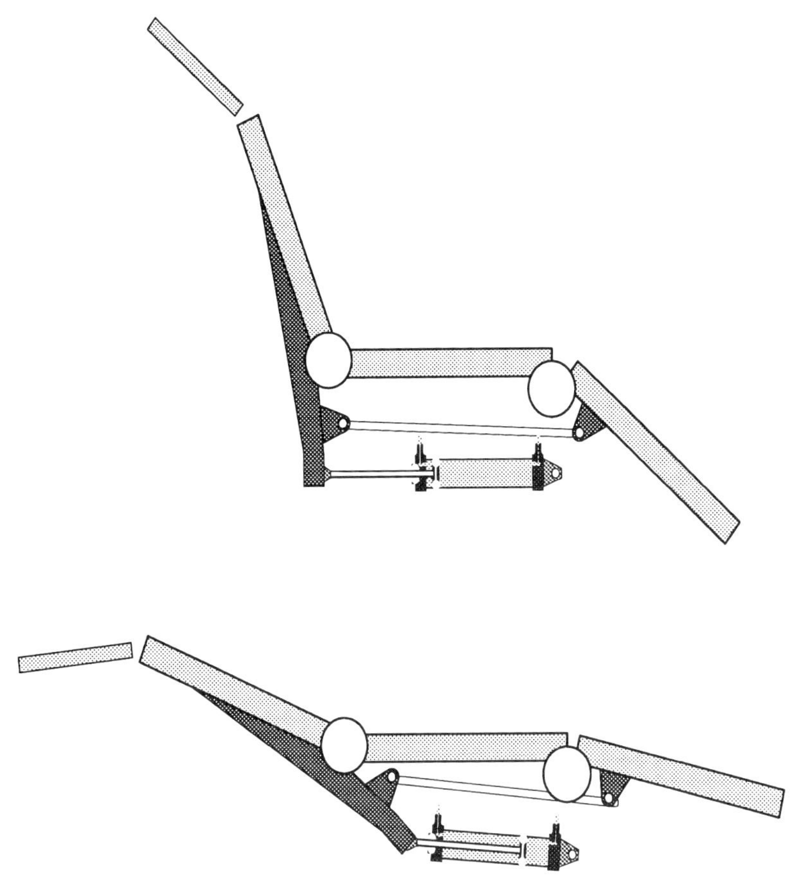

Fig. 9. Hydraulic control of back-rest.

Upholstery

The upholstery of dental chairs suffers severe use and needs to be tough and well-looked after if it is to survive for a useful period. Most dental chairs are covered with vinyl over foam plastic. The vinyl should be cleaned regularly with an appropriate vinyl cleaner which will maintain the plasticisers in the covering and postpone cracking and splitting of the surface.

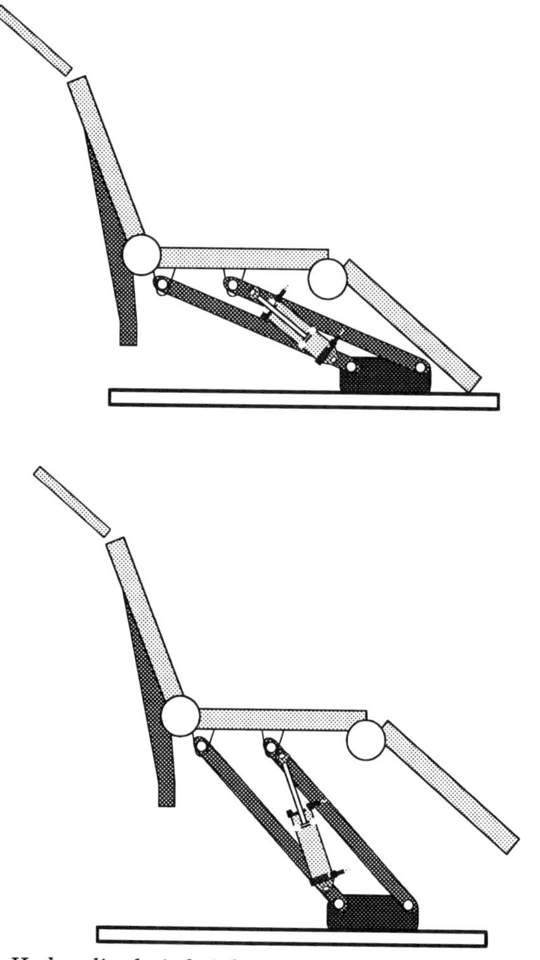

Fig. 10. Hydraulic chair height control.

Care must be taken when disinfectants are used. Certain disinfectants will cause rapid perishing of the vinyl surface. The specific instructions of the chair manufacturer for disinfection should be followed.

There has been a fashion in covering dental chairs with fabrics such as velvet, apparently to decrease the clinical atmosphere of the operatory. Such fabrics do not lend themselves well to cleaning and the avoidance of cross-infection.

Dental lights

Effective lighting is essential to efficient, stress-free operative dentistry. Lighting needs to be intense at the site of operation but must be combined with strong ambient lighting. Intense light localised to the area of operation against a dim background creates strong contrast which may be extremely tiring as the operator's eyes are forced into repetitive adaptation between the two intensity levels.

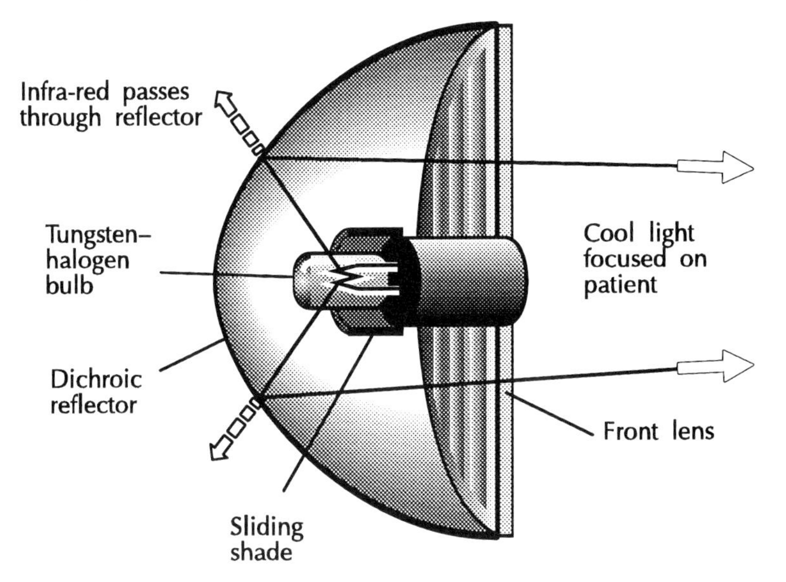

Fig. 11. Operating light.

The operating light should provide an even illumination with cool light. This should be restricted to the operating area and should not shine in the patients eyes. Cool light is visible light with a low infra-red content. Hot wire filament bulbs of all types produce a considerable amount of infra-red heat in addition to the visible component. This should be removed by means of filters. A dichroic reflector is the most common method of achieving this *(Fig. 11)*. The reflector reflects visible light but is transparent to infra-red. Only the cool visible light is directed onto the patient's face.

The best light for the operative area is that from quartz–halogen bulbs. These devices allow appropriate focusing to give an even illumination combined with masking so that the patients eyes are not illuminated.

When a normal incandescent electric light bulb operates the metal filament vaporises slowly. This vapour is deposited on the inside of the glass envelope of the bulb and gradually reduces the light output. Furthermore, as the metal is lost the filament becomes thinned. Localised thinning causes that area of the filament to run hotter and hence vaporise more rapidly. Damage to this area of the filament accelerates and the filament eventually blows. Running such a bulb at higher temperatures results in an increased light output at a better colour temperature but also leads to an extremely short life.

Tungsten–halogen bulbs consist of a tungsten filament in a quartz envelope filled with halogen vapour. As tungsten evaporates from the filament it combines with the halogen vapour and is redeposited onto the filament by a further chemical reaction. This means that the filament can operate at a far higher temperature than a conventional bulb without the bulb blackening from the deposition of metal on the inside of the glass envelope.

Special care needs to be taken when changing a tungsten–halogen bulb. Firstly, because the bulb runs so much hotter than a conventional bulb, adequate time must be allowed for the glass envelope to cool. Secondly, the new bulb must under no circumstances be handled directly. Sodium from the skin is absorbed into the quartz envelope and will combine with the halogen vapour, reducing the efficiency and life of the bulb. Most tungsten–halogen bulbs are supplied packed with a cardboard sleeve over the envelope which allows the bulb to be handled. When the bulb is in place in its holder the sleeve is removed.

Variable brightness may be an advantage but care must be taken to select a system which does not affect the colour balance of the light. Units which alter the light intensity by varying the voltage to the bulb are not desirable because the colour of the light will alter significantly with the level of illumination. As the voltage is reduced, to lessen the light output, the temperature of the bulb filament is reduced and the colour of the light given off tends to become redder. As the temperature is raised the light becomes blue. Electronic control using thyristor switching is less desirable because this also has an effect on the filament temperature and hence colour balance and may introduce an added stroboscopic effect if the switching frequency is too low.

The solution is to use a light which maintains the bulb filament at a constant temperature and alters the light output by sliding a masking shade into the light pathway. Such lights can be used for shade assessment for aesthetic dentistry at any illumination level.

Colour perception

Great care is needed to select appropriate lighting when shades are being matched for aesthetic restorations. Probably the best light to use is a colour-balanced tungsten–halogen unit of the type described above. Fluorescent light is rich in green and peaks sharply over several areas of the colour spectrum and is grossly unsuitable for colour and shade selection.

Fibre-optic handpieces

Light can be directed down a handpiece to illuminate the bur using fibre-optic light guides. Today, both turbines and motor/handpiece combinations are available with fibre-optic illumination.

In most systems a miniature low-voltage quartz–halogen bulb is located in the shank of the handpiece and the light guided through the head casing to emerge alongside the coolant spray. Many operators find fibre-optic handpieces invaluable. Restrictions on acceptable sterilising methods are found with some models.

One handpiece lighting system available today uses a complete annular light source emerging from a ring lens around the bur. This gives genuine shadow-free illumination of the operating area.

CHAPTER 2

Investigative Systems

Investigative systems are those associated with the acquisition of information relating to normal structures or pathological conditions. The most important investigative technology in clinical dentistry is radiography.

X-rays

X-ray diagnosis or radiology provides a major mode of diagnosis in dentistry. However because of the hazards of radiation it is necessary to minimise the exposure to the patient and operator. To do this effectively it is necessary to understand how X-ray systems work, where an X-ray examination can be of value and where other investigative methods could provide equal information.

Generation of X-rays

The target is set in a copper block to achieve cooling. In the higher power X-ray sets which are necessary for large-film views, the target is built as a cone which can be rotated rapidly in use to prevent the localised build-up of heat in a static target. A small focal spot is desirable to ensure that the X-ray beam produces a sharp image.

X-rays are generated by the action of electrons striking a tungsten target *(Fig. 12)*. The electrons are produced by heating a metal wire filament in a vacuum. These form as a cloud clustering around the wire and are then accelerated away by attracting them to a high voltage. This forms a beam of electrons.

The accelerated electron beam is focused to a small spot on a target of tungsten. This is known as the focal spot. As the electrons hit the tungsten atoms they cause the electrons of the target atom to rise to a higher energy level or orbital. As these electrons drop back to their original levels they re-radiate the energy with a different wavelength, in this case X-rays *(Fig. 13)*.

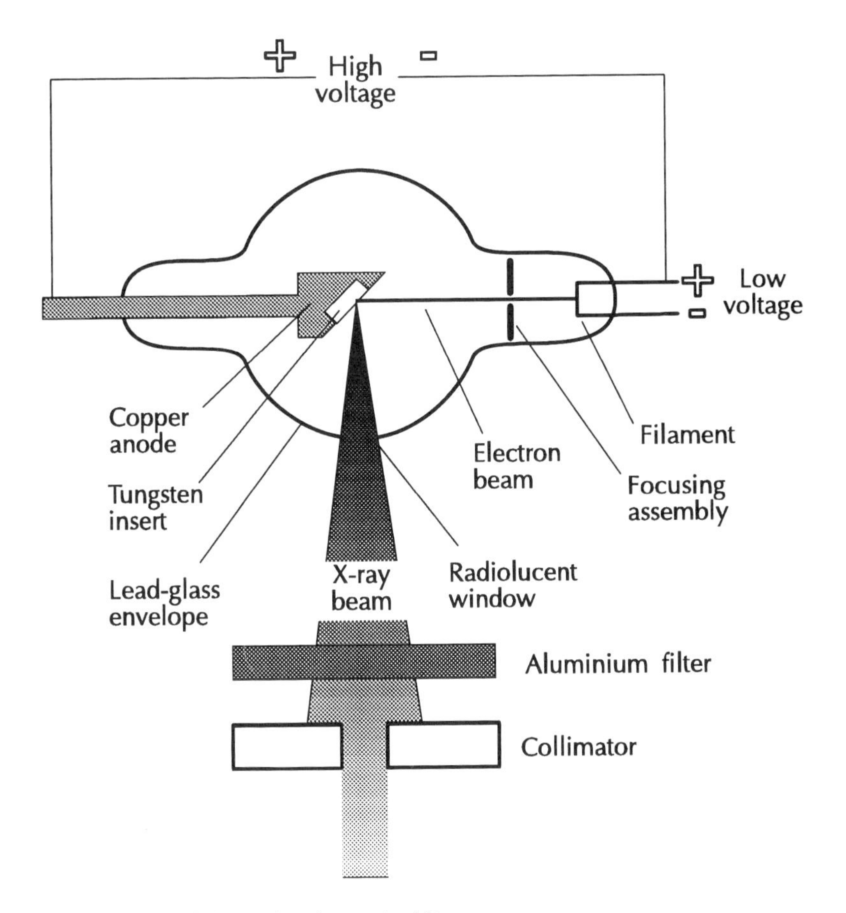

Fig. 12. Schematic of a typical X-ray set.

The X-ray energy given off can be characterised in two main parameters, the frequency and the energy delivered *(Fig. 14)*. The frequency is dependant upon the accelerating voltage, a higher voltage producing X-rays of higher frequency or higher photon energy. A low frequency has low penetrating power and is absorbed by the skin and soft tissues. It is necessary to use a frequency of sufficient penetrating power to penetrate through teeth.

The high voltage is generated by a transformer. The voltage delivered to the X-ray tube may be alternating current (a.c.) or direct current (d.c.). There is a considerable difference in the output of the two systems. The voltage in the a.c. system will rise and fall from peak to zero during each cycle. The frequency of the

X-rays produced will rise and fall accordingly. Direct current generators maintain a constant voltage and a correspondingly constant X-ray spectrum.

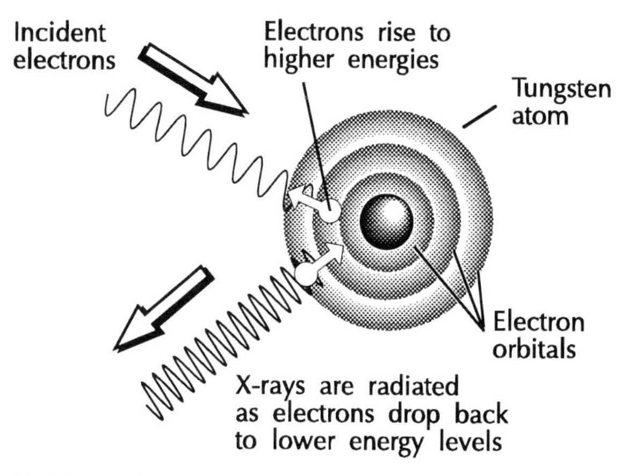

Fig. 13. The production of X-rays.

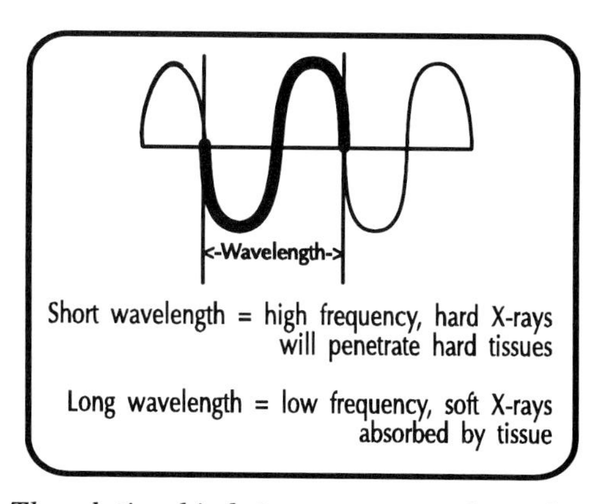

Fig. 14. The relationship between energy and wavelength.

The power output of the tube is determined by the current flowing through the heated filament and is usually expressed in mA. Most dental sets operate with tube currents in the range 5–20 mA.

The tube and high voltage transformer are encased in a steel housing which is mounted on an articulated arm to allow it to be manipulated about the patient *(Fig. 15)*.

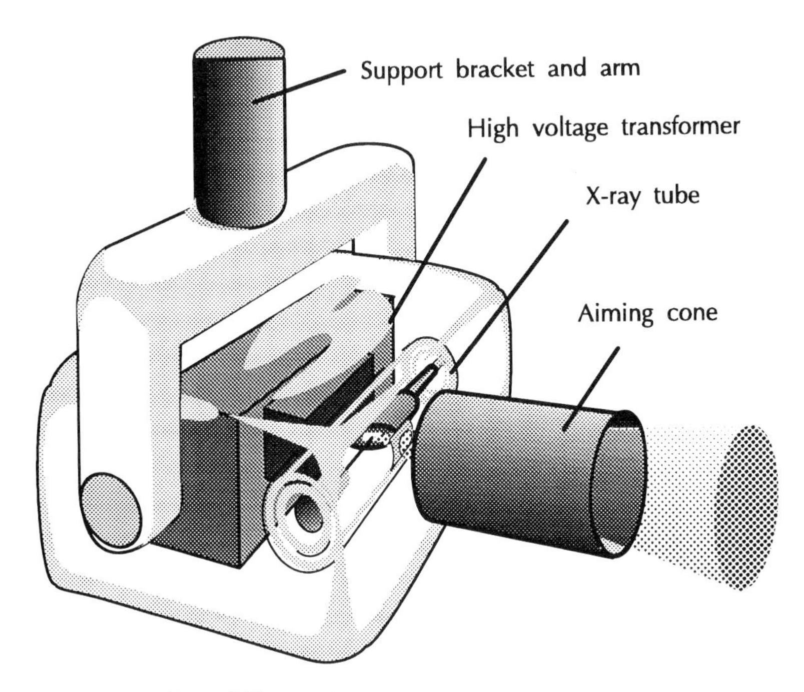

Fig. 15. Dental X-ray set.

An accurate timer is essential in the construction of an X-ray set and nowadays this is usually electronic. For safety, a pilot light and accompanying audio tone should indicate when X-rays are being produced and generation should cease immediately the operator releases the exposure button. The overall output of a tube can be indicated by multiplying the tube current by the time and is expressed as milliampere seconds (mAs).

The whole tube head is manufactured with shielding to ensure that the only place where X-rays escape is the primary beam and that no leakage occurs in any other direction.

Standard dental X-ray set

For most applications, a standard dental X-ray set should have an accelerating voltage of at least 70 kV. This will provide a relatively 'hard' X-ray beam of high frequency. This will penetrate teeth effectively. X-rays with lower frequencies from a source less than 50 kV are not of lesser diagnostic value and are absorbed in the tissues rather than contributing effectively to the radiographic image.

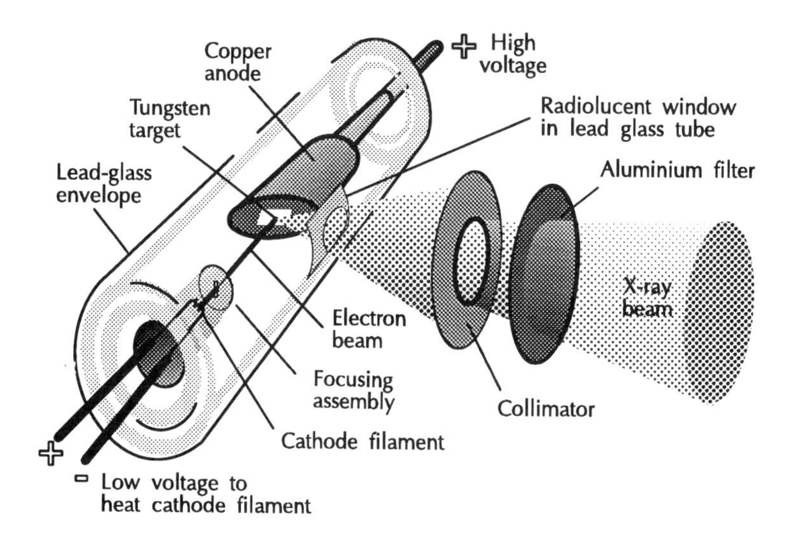

Fig. 16. A dental X-ray tube head.

Fig. 16 shows a typical dental X-ray unit. The X-ray beam from the tube is filtered through an aluminium filter to remove the lower frequency X-rays, or soft X-rays, which are of no value because they would only be absorbed by the tissues rather than penetrating through to the film. A narrow beam is produced by collimating the X-rays through an aperture in a steel or lead plate.

The standard dental X-ray set must be manoeuvred and angled through a considerable space around the patient's head. This is accomplished by attaching the set to a counterbalanced, articulated arm which supports the tube head and enables it to be moved rapidly and angled accurately. It is important that while the tube can be moved easily it must remain stationary when released. This requires very careful adjustment of the support arms and accurate alignment so that the main column sits in the true vertical.

Modern tubes move the focal spot to the back of the tube-head by projecting the X-rays through the centre of the transformer which moves to the front of the tube *(Fig. 17)*.

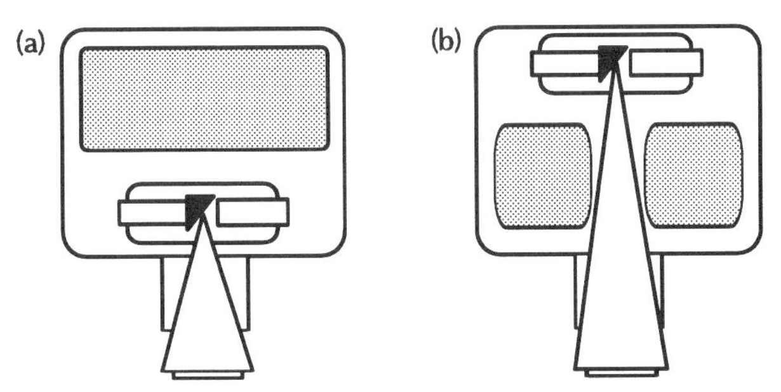

Fig. 17. (a) Standard X-ray tube. (b) Toroidal transformer allows repositioning of the X-ray tube and greater target–film distance with less beam divergence.

A radical change in transformer design is necessary to allow this and a toroidal design is adopted. The X-ray beam can be projected though the aperture in this doughnut-shaped structure. This tube-head design produces a beam with less divergence than the traditional design, giving a film image with less distortion due to enlargement. Also the relative size of the focal spot is reduced giving a higher resolution image.

Panoramic systems

Many systems are available now which allow the operator to take a full-mouth scan of the patient. Several systems have been developed but those which are now in common use rely mainly on the principle of the tomogram. One system of interest reversed the normal film-tube orientation by placing the X-ray tube intra-orally and projecting the image onto a screened film held against the patient's face in a flexible packet.

In tomographic systems, the object to be radiographed is kept still whilst the X-ray tube and the film are moved in synchronism about a common axis *(Fig. 18)*.

The action of the machine is illustrated in *Fig. 19*. A slit collimator at the tube end forms a thin vertical beam of X-rays which are further collimated by a narrow slit in a metal screen which covers the film. The film moves slowly past this slit in order to build up an image.

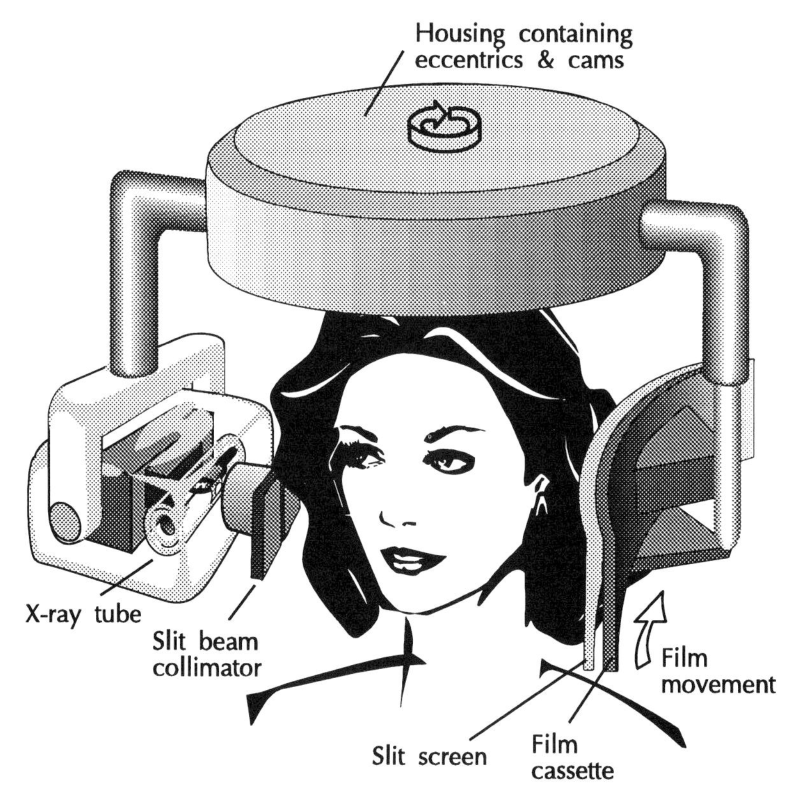

Fig. 18. Basic layout of a panoramic X-ray machine.

The concept of the tomogram is to move the film and the X-ray beam relative to the subject in such a way that the movement of the film and the plane of of the structures to be viewed is synchronised. At the plane of view the movement of the film relative to the movement of the tube around the patient will be such that the image cast of the plane of view will be stationary on the film. Structures on either side of the plane of cut will move at a greater rate and this movement will blur them out. The system is analogous to the movement of a printing press. Provided the paper is moved across the printing drum at the same speed, an image will be transferred and the print will be clear. If the paper is moved faster or slower than the surface of the drum then the inked image which is transferred will be smeared or blurred. In the panoramic X-ray machine, as the device rotates around the patient, the film is counter-rotated so that it moves past the structures to be imaged like the paper across the printing drum. All structures outside this plane will be moving relative to the film and will be smeared or blurred across the film such that they become indistinct hazes compared with the sharp image from the focal plane.

The whole tube-film complex orbits around a central axis which is related to the film rotation and film-tube movement. This axis is made to follow the line of the jaw as it orbits around the patient. This complicated movement *(Fig. 20)* is operated by a series of cams and levers in a housing above the patient. The patient is positioned correctly within the geometry of the machine by either biting on a mouth block or by placing the chin on a chin-rest. The radiographer is assisted in positioning the patient within this geometry by a series of light lines which are projected onto the face.

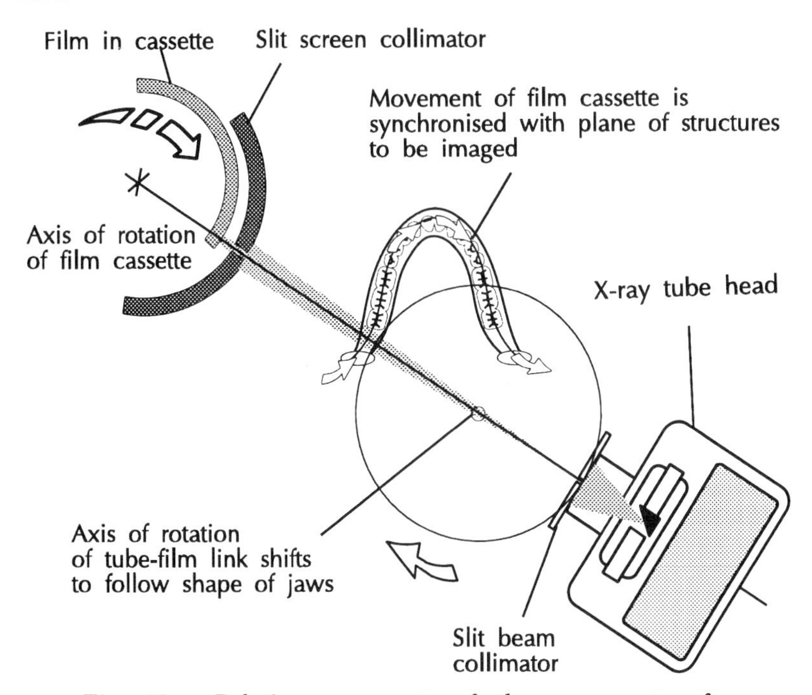

Fig. 19. Relative movements of the components of a panoramic X-ray machine.

The X-ray tube in panoramic and cephalometric sets requires a greater range of output energy and this may be selectable between 50 and 110 kV.

Variations on the configuration illustrated are produced. Some sets use just two or three points of rotation of the film and tube around the patient and some accomplish this by actually moving the patient laterally in a chair from one axis point to the other.

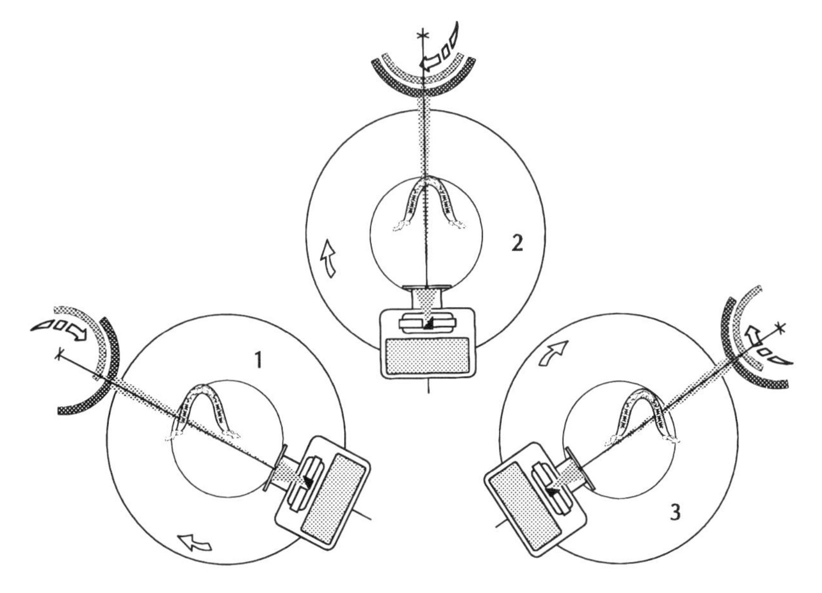

Fig. 20. Path of movement of a panoramic X-ray unit.

Films and screens

The most common method of recording an image from an X-ray examination is to use a photographic film. A latent image is created in a silver halide emulsion and this is changed chemically into deposits of colloidal silver during development, thus producing a visible image. Photographic film is sensitive to a range of electromagnetic radiation ranging from infra-red to X-rays. A number of techniques are used to maximise the clarity of the image whilst minimising the exposure of the patient to radiation.

Twin emulsion films

Whilst standard photographic film is only coated on one side with a sensitive emulsion, X-ray film is usually coated on both sides. In this way the X-ray beam produces two exposures and the images are coincident and summate when viewed. The addition of one image over the next increases the contrast ratio of the film dramatically and a reduced exposure time can be used. This reduces the dose of radiation absorbed by the patient.

Intensifying screens

Like other forms of electromagnetic radiation, X-rays can cause fluorescence in certain materials. When X-rays hit atoms of calcium tungstate they cause electrons to rise into higher energy states. As these electrons drop back to their stable lower energy state they release the energy they gained from the X-rays at a different wavelength, that of visible light. If such a material is coated onto a carrying screen, the screen will glow with a clear image when placed in front of an X-ray set. This is principle of intensifying screens. A twin emulsion film is sandwiched between two intensifying screens inside an aluminium cassette. When exposed to X-rays, the beam can pass through the radiolucent aluminium case, causing the first screen to glow and exposing the film to a visible light image. The two layers of film emulsion are then exposed directly by the beam which then encounters the second intensifying screen and again produces another copy of the visible light image. In this way, the image produced in the film is intensified greatly.

Whilst calcium tungstate was used in early screens, the most dramatic fluorescence can be obtained with rare-earth mineral screens and these, though far more expensive, are replacing the older type and reducing the radiation exposure of patients even further.

Automatic developers

Various machines for the automated development of radiographs have been devised. The most popular of the larger throughput systems utilises a series of rubber rollers and guides to route the film through the system *(Fig. 21)*.

The film is guided sequentially through the developer, a wash or stop bath, the fixer and then a final wash. The developer develops the image by causing the precipitation of colloidal silver from the silver salts within the gelatin emulsion of the film. The stop bath is an acid which arrests the action of the developer and prevents it from carrying over and contaminating the fixative. The fix bath removes all unused silver salts and renders the silver image permanent. The wash stage removes unused fixative to prevent the image fading from continued reaction with the fixative. In many machines hot air is blown over the film to dry it before it is delivered out of the unit.

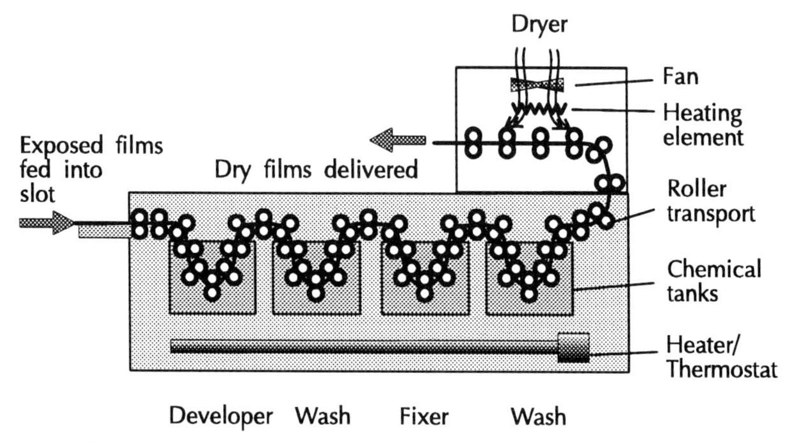

Fig. 21. A typical automatic roller processor for radiographs.

The roller system has the advantage of continuous processing with minimal contamination across solutions. The only chemicals to pass from one bath to another are those retained on the surface and in the gelatin of the film being processed. However continuous development means a gradual exhaustion of the chemicals and replenishment is needed. This may be automatic or manual. A small quantity of concentrated developer is added to the first bath at intervals after a predetermined area of film has been processed.

Automatic processors need attentive maintenance to retain efficient operation. The chemicals need to be changed regularly and the whole unit cleaned out.

Cheaper automatic processors are available which use a dip and dunk system of film transport. Films are loaded into a carrying cassette which is then lifted and dipped into the various solutions sequentially. Some of these systems have to cycle the cassette through the system before they are capable of receiving further films.

Xeroradiography

Wet-developed silver halide films have provided the major method of image recording in X-ray systems for years. However recent times have seen the development of a dry-film system which provides almost instant high resolution views. This is known as xeroradiography.

Xeroradiography projects the X-ray beam onto a plate made out of selenium which has been given a large electrostatic charge. Where the X-ray beam can penetrate and hit the film-plate the charge is lost. In this way an electrostatic image of the X-ray can be created. Development consists of spreading a toner powder over the surface of the plate, transferring it to a piece of carrier film and then melting it on to create the image. The high cost of the initial equipment purchase together with the relative complexity of machine servicing has limited the uptake of this technology. Xeroradiographic images provide an increased level of contrast and demonstrate edge effects between areas of high contrast. This can lead to misleading interpretation of the film by operators not familiar with these image effects. However, the edge enhancement effects together with the speed of operation make the system extremely useful for endodontic canal-length determination.

Contrast radiography

Many structures do not have sufficient difference in radiodensity from the surrounding tissues to display themselves within the contrast limitations of conventional radiography. However, it is sometimes possible to reveal such structures by coating them with a radiopaque dye to increase the contrast. This technique is known as contrast radiography.

A good example of its use in dentistry is sialography, the examination of the duct structure of salivary glands. A liquid containing barium is injected into the orifice of the salivary gland to be investigated and when the duct structure has been back-filled fully, a radiograph is taken revealing the boundaries of dye penetration. This may disclose pathoses such as duct stricture or calculi, or may indicate the presence of a space-occupying growth.

CCD imagers

The breakthrough which allowed the development of the miniature television cameras which are built into the ubiquitous camcorder beloved of tourists was the charge-coupled-device (CCD) imaging unit. It is this device which has been exploited in electronic imaging systems for dental radiographs, referred to by one manufacturer as 'radiovisiography'*(Fig. 22)*.

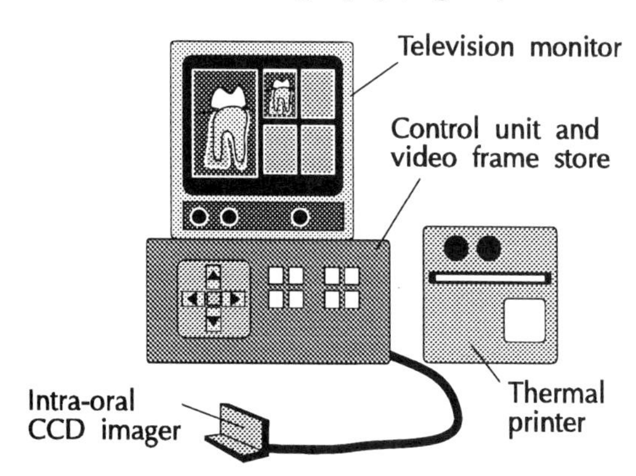

Fig. 22. Radiovisiography unit.

The CCD imager is a solid state microchip which is sensitive to light. The X-ray image is formed on a phosphorescent screen which is used in place of the conventional film. This screen converts the X-ray image to light, which is channelled to the tiny CCD device through a converging fibre-optic bundle.

The CCD imager can be made small enough to substitute for a periapical-size X-ray film *(Fig. 23)*. This is placed behind the tooth to be imaged and exposed in the manner of a conventional radiograph. However, the image is recorded electronically and stored in a solid-state memory known as a digital frame store. It can then be displayed on a television monitor or recorded onto magnetic media such as a computer disk.

The system has a number of advantages over photochemical systems. Firstly, it requires a reduced dosage of X-rays. Secondly, the image is effectively instantaneous. However, there is a penalty to be paid. The resolution of current systems is substantially less than that of X-ray film and this may limit its use.

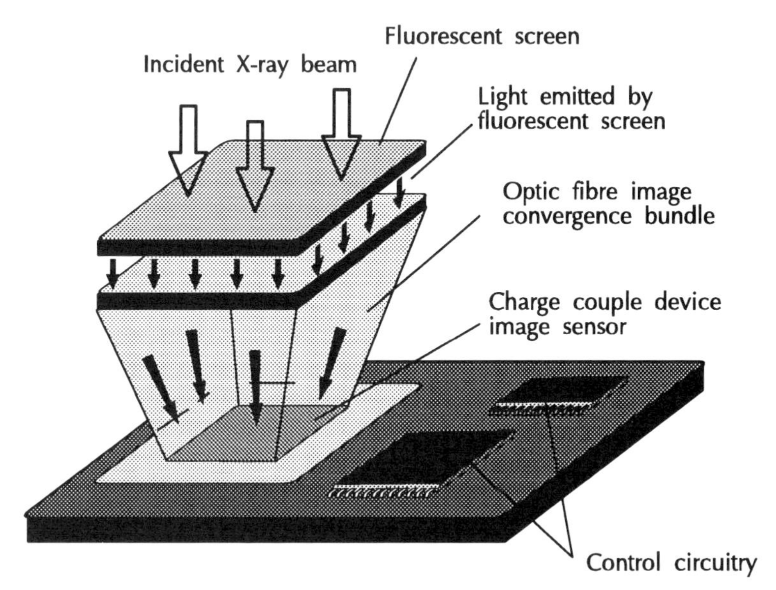

Fig. 23. Radiovisiography sensor.

Computerised axial tomography

Computerised axial tomography (CAT) revolutionised radiography by adding the third dimension to the views obtained. CAT scans produce a three-dimensional image in the true sense. Accurate and detailed transverse slices can be reconstructed. The system consists of an X-ray tube which produces a narrow beam of radiation which is measured electronically by a detector. The output from the detector is proportional to the absorption of X-radiation by the intervening tissues. The tube and detector scan across the body to produce a raster image. The tube and detector then swing to another angle and repeat the scan. By analysing the variation in radiodensity from several angles, the density of any point can be calculated. From this information, a three-dimensional lattice can be constructed by a computer and displayed on a television monitor. Computer manipulation of the data can create dramatic and highly informative three-dimensional views of the structures examined.

Magnetic resonance imaging

Magnetic resonance imaging (MRI) is a very exciting area of development. This method relies purely on a magnetic phenomenon of water dipoles and is non-invasive and totally safe. The constraints of radiation exposure which apply to X-radiation are of no significance in this respect.

When water is exposed to a large magnetic field the dipoles of the water flip into alignment with the field. When the field is switched off the dipoles flip back to their original random state but in the process of each action a minute level of radio waves are released. By detecting the radio waves and their origin, the structure of the containing tissue may be examined. Extremely high resolution views can be obtained. With a compromise of resolution some limited real-time movement can be achieved. The unique feature of the machine is that it is able to show hard and soft tissues with ease on the same film.

MRI has a wide range of applications in medicine. For example, the dynamics of blood flow through the heart can be seen clearly. In dentistry, the system is useful in maxillo-facial surgery for the examination of tissues for tumours and for investigating the health of the temporomandibular joint. However it has the great drawback of a considerable initial expense and a high resolution image can take some time to record. Its use is limited to specialist centres in major hospitals.

Safety standards

A discussion of regulations relating to radiation safety is beyond the scope of this book and the reader is directed to the local regulations under which he must operate. However, some general guidelines can be provided.

Firstly, X-ray examination must only be undertaken when there is a clear need. One of the best ways of limiting diagnostic radiation is to ensure that the diagnostic system is running effectively and that repeat films are a rarity. Trained staff and well-maintained equipment are essential. The developing and processing system must be running as efficiently as possible to ensure that an effective image can be obtained from the least radiation exposure.

Compensating for inadequate processing by increasing the exposure times is inexcusable.

Local regulations specify the minimum distance from the tube to clinical personnel during operation but in all circumstances no-one but the patient must be exposed to the primary beam.

Electrical

Endodontic impedance measurement

Root canal treatment of teeth requires a knowledge of the length of the pulp space so that the entire void can be prepared then obturated fully by the root filling. Determination of canal length by taking a radiograph with a radiopaque marker of known length in the canal is the most common and accepted method but is not perfect. Curves and distortions may lead to a non-linear image. Furthermore, the actual point to be located in the measurement, the apical constriction, is not visible radiographically but has to be deduced from surrounding structures. The overall accuracy of this method has been estimated at 80%. The method lacks convenience although the use of radiovisiography (see page 28) has reduced the time delay and inconvenience of length-determining radiographs.

Impedance measuring devices are an alternative or adjunct to such X-ray techniques. The electrical properties of the pulp space vary along its length and this change can be measured. The specific property which is monitored is the electrical impedance. Impedance is the resistance of a structure to the passage of an alternating current. It is the a.c. equivalent of d.c. resistance and is a function of the resistance, inductance and capacitance of the circuit.

The patient is grounded to the earth return of the testing device *(Fig. 24)*. A test electrode is attached to an endodontic file which is inserted into the root canal. As the file approaches the apical constriction a significant change in electrical impedance occurs and this is used to indicate its position. The output from the device may be in the form of a meter reading or a series of coloured lights. Several devices use an audio tone to indicate when the apical constriction has been reached.

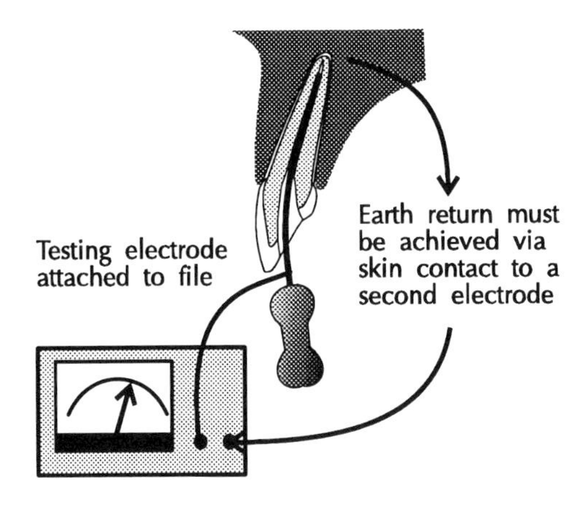

Fig. 24. Electrical determination of root canal length.

Impedance measuring devices are not without limitations. Electrolytes in the root canal such as pus or irrigants can affect the readings to the point of incoherence. When used correctly some of these devices provide an acceptable level of accuracy but there is considerable variation between designs.

Caries impedance tester

When enamel and dentine are demineralised by dental caries their electrical properties change. The electrical impedance of the tooth can be measured at the base of the fissure system to detect the presence of caries. Though the change in impedance which occurs is not great, there is a difference between carious and normal teeth. Caries-detecting meters are available but are relatively insensitive. They are not capable of determining small changes or the true extent of lesions.

Pulp testers

Often it is necessary to determine whether the pulp in a tooth is alive or dead. Methods of testing include the application of heat or cold stimuli to the surface of the tooth and stimulation of the pulp electrically. The electrical apparatus for testing the pulp is depicted in *Fig. 25*. The voltage from a battery is raised by a small electronic circuit and a pulsed, high voltage direct current is delivered to the tooth. The current flow can be regulated by means of a control dial on the outside of the casing although some modern devices ramp the current up automatically at a fixed rate. The current is delivered to the surface enamel of the tooth to be tested via a conductive rubber pad. An indicator lamp usually lights to indicate that the tester is operating but does not necessarily indicate that a current is flowing. An earth return to the pulp tester is necessary and can be achieved by either direct skin contact through the hand of the operator or by a second electrode. The former method is found in many testers but the circuit is broken if the operator is wearing gloves. A false negative result may be obtained inadvertently if the operator is not aware of this problem, although at very high voltages positive tests may be obtained. Similarly, large metallic restorations in a tooth or highly insulative porcelain crowns can lead to false readings due to locally altered conduction pathways. Bipolar pulp testers, which apply an electrode to either side of the tooth to be tested, have been used experimentally to advantage.

In use, the unit is pressed against undamaged enamel on the labial surface of the tooth to be tested and the control dial turned slowly to raise the current until the patient is just aware of an uncomfortable sensation in the tooth. The threshold of stimulation occurs typically at currents between 1 and 20 micro-amps. The resistance of the tooth ranges from around 1 Megohm to 60 Megohms. whilst the capacitance varies from 25 pF to 100 pF. Voltages in excess of 200 V may be necessary to reach the threshold of stimulation. Some pulp testers are capable of delivering 800 V. The output of the unit may vary in polarity, frequency and wave-form as well as voltage and current and this will alter the threshold of stimulation.

Whenever possible a test is made on the tooth contra-lateral to the one being examined. This acts as a control and gives a reference level for sensitivity if it is not itself damaged or heavily restored.

Thermal and electrical tests are usually accompanied by a radiographic examination for changes associated with an apical response.

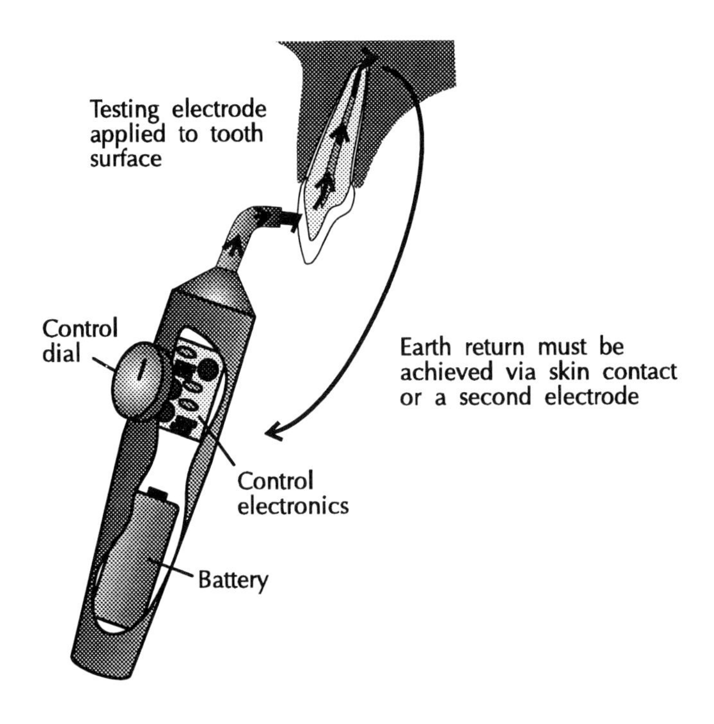

Fig. 25. Operation of a pulp tester.

Thermal and electrical tests are usually accompanied by a radiographic examination for changes associated with an apical response.

Whilst the majority of pulp testers are designed for total electrical safety, the use of electronic equipment which produces high voltages and pulsed currents is not appropriate on patients with unshielded pace-makers.

Optical aids

Many operative procedures may be implemented with increased efficiency and ease if magnification is used. Examples range from the detection of caries to the location of root canal orifices. In the laboratory additional magnification is of great help in such procedures as die trimming.

The simplest form of magnification is the magnifying glass. Small magnifying glasses can be mounted on an arm in front of a spectacle frame or can be worn as a visor from a head band and will give a useful magnification of up to x2. These magnifiers give magnification at the expense of having to get closer to the subject. This may be acceptable in the dental laboratory but is less so in the clinical area.

The distance between the operator and the working site can only be increased if telescope optical are used. The simplest form of telescopic magnification is the Galilean telescope. This uses a concave lens for the eyepiece and a convex lens for the objective. This is the system used in many simple binoculars such as opera glasses. This works well but gives a limited magnification in the region of x2. To achieve higher magnification it is necessary to use a system of complex convex lenses in the manner of an astromomical telescope. This can provide magnifications well beyond that necessary for any clinical dental or laboratory procedure. However, a problem arises with this optical system in that reversal and inversion of the image occur between the objective lens and the eyepiece. This must be corrected if the system is going to be of any use. Conventional binoculars do this by inserting two correcting prisms into the optical pathway which reverse and invert the image to restore its orientation. These correcting prisms are usually large and clumsy and are known as porro prisms. A much more compact system has been developed and is known as the roof prism system. This is used in compact binoculars and opera glasses and has been adopted for most dental and surgical loupes. The system is illustrated in *Fig. 26*. The prisms are entirely coaxial in the optical axis of the lenses and are much lighter and neater than porro prism designs. However, they are much more difficult and critical to manufacture and in consequence command a much greater price.

A further stage on from the optical loupe is the operating microscope. This uses a similar optical system to the one described but the binoculars are mounted on an adjustable stand instead of being worn from a headband. Operating microscopes designed specifically for dentistry are available. The operating microscope usually includes a lighting source which is coaxial with the field of view. This provides the operator with shadow-free lighting of the operating field. Additionally, a television camera may be mounted into the unit to allow an audience to view the operating field through the eyes of the operator.

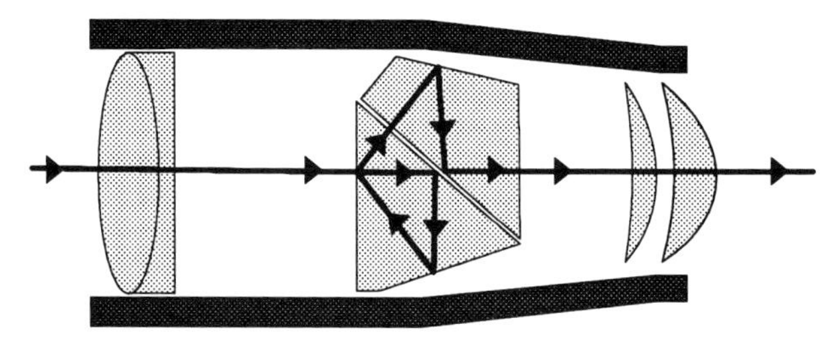

Fig. 26. Optical loupes of roof prism design.

Fibre-optic transillumination

Fibre-optic transillumination is a useful adjunct in diagnostic procedures including caries detection, crack detection, etc. A small diameter (approx. 2 mm) fibre-optic bundle is illuminated by a suitable light source, ideally quartz–halogen. The operation of fibre-optic bundles is described on page 79. The entire unit may be hand-held or the light source may be mains-powered and bench mounted. Some dental units include fibre-optic diagnostic lights in the instrument delivery unit.

CHAPTER 3

Rotary Instrumentation

The principle of contra-angulation

A straight handpiece is the simplest and most stable design for rotary instruments but has very little use in the mouth because of limitation of access. For most purposes it is necessary to have the axis of rotation of the cutting bur in axial alignment with the tooth. This means that the shaft of the handpiece has to be at an angle to the shank *(Fig. 27)*.

The simplest way to do this is to turn the drive through 90°. There is a problem with this configuration in that it is difficult and unwieldy to handle. When a bur cuts against a tooth it will produce a displacing force 90° to the axis of rotation. If the bur can form a lever arm with the handpiece then it will tend to rotate

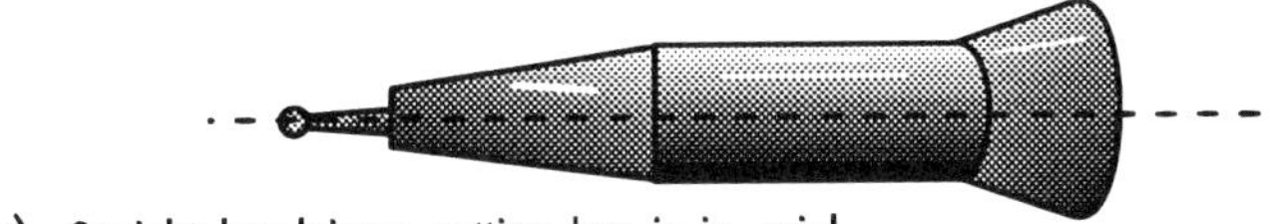

(a) Straight handpiece: cutting bur is in axial alignment with the handpiece

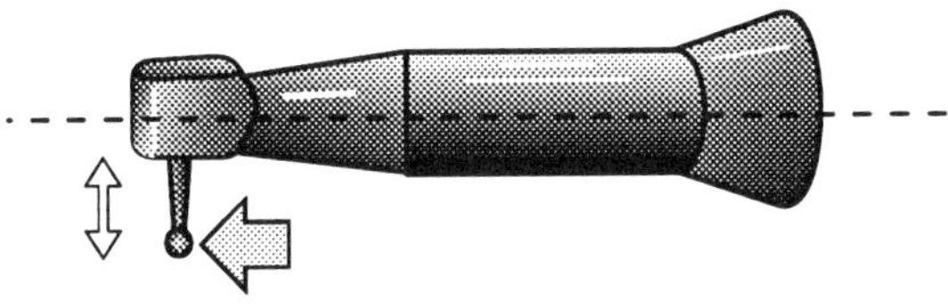

(b) Right angle handpiece: bur is offset from handpiece axis, forming a lever arm and leading to instability

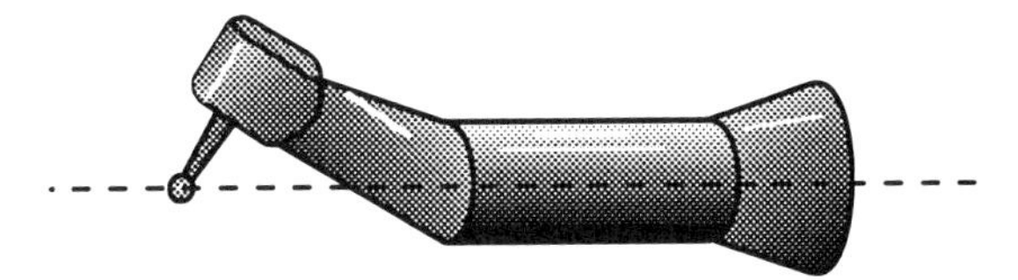

(c) Contra-angle handpiece: cutting bur is aligned with the axis of the handpiece making a controllable, stable system.

Fig. 27. Contra-angulation.

the whole handpiece. This is unstable and difficult to resist.

The principle of contra-angulation introduces a second angle into the handpiece to return the tip of the bur to the long axis of the handpiece. This removes the lever arm and the consequent rotation of the handpiece. Contra-angulation provides both access and stability to the instrument.

Air turbines have a high speed and low torque and are not capable of producing the high lateral forces of a motor and handpiece. Consequently, contra-angulation in turbines is attenuated to a greater or lesser extent depending upon the design.

Air turbine

The air turbine has become the instrument of greatest importance in operative dentistry. Its invention revolutionised the preparation of teeth for restorations. Early attempts at achieving high speed rotation were not made in an effort to improve the speed of cut but to improve patient comfort through the reduced perception of vibration at high frequency. However, the increased ease and speed of cut were the features which led to the development and marketing of the device.

The first dental drills to reach speeds above 100 000 rpm were geared up handpieces running from conventional electric motors. Later, water turbines were tried and met with some success. Hydraulic turbines are capable of very high torque but not extremely high speeds. The air turbine provided the ultimate solution.

Dental air turbines are capable of achieving extremely high rotational speed up to 500 000 rpm. Higher speeds are possible but offer little advantage and many disadvantages as limits of mechanical stress and wear are soon reached. Additionally, the lack of tactile appreciation of cutting with turbines running at such speeds makes preparations very difficult.

A number of problems arise when turbines are operating at speeds in excess of 250 000 rpm. Firstly, the wear on the support bearings is very great indeed. Some handpieces overcome this problem by suspending the rotating turbine and cutting bur in air bearings. In principle, these should last forever, but the lateral forces of free-hand cutting can cause the bearing to crash as the air cushion is overpowered. The life of such handpieces depends very much on the skill and care with which the operator uses the handpiece. An understanding and effective operator may get many years of service out of a single set of bearings, whereas the less careful can wreck such a turbine during the execution of a single procedure.

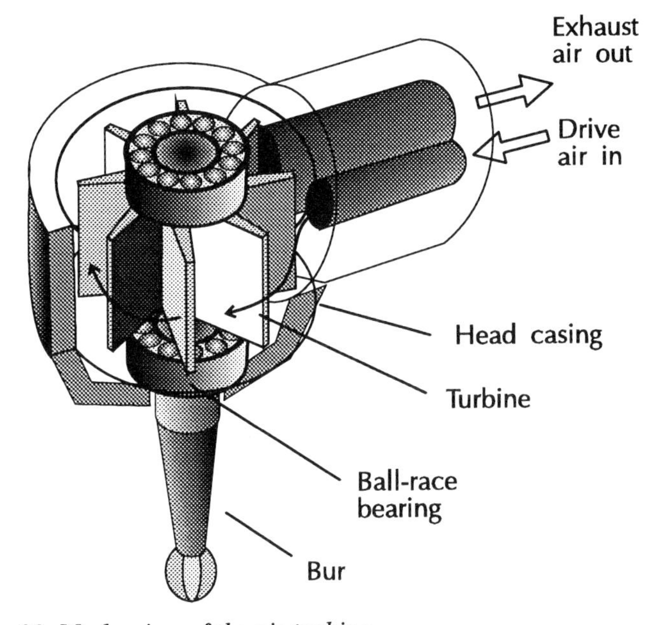

Fig. 28. Mechanism of the air turbine.

In order to overcome the problem of lateral forces causing bearing crash and hence reducing the effective torque of a handpiece, many modern designs utilise miniature ball-races to suspend the rotor *(Fig. 28)*. These are finely engineered from extremely hard alloys and provide an excellent compromise. They are very much less susceptible to the ravages of the less sensitive operator and can provide higher effective torque because they cannot be stalled at the bearing. They will only stall when the torque resistance is greater than the air pressure feeding the rotor.

Air turbine handpieces with air-suspension bearings require a supply air pressure of 0.35 to 0.5 MPa (50 to 70 psi). Ball-race bearing handpieces operate at a pressure of 0.2 to 0.35 MPa (30 to 50 psi). It is important to measure the supply pressure at the end of the handpiece tubing and not within the supply unit because the pressure can drop significantly in the connecting hose. Furthermore the pressure gauge should be inserted at the coupling into the handpiece so that dynamic air-pressure is measured and not static pressure which may be considerably greater.

Although air turbines may have a free-running speed of 250–500 000 rpm, this is reduced rapidly under load. Speeds of around 100 000 rpm are common when the bur is actually cutting.

Considerable heat is generated when an air turbine is cutting teeth. This heat has to be removed rapidly from the cutting site. A water spray alone is inadequate for this purpose, a copious aerosol is far more efficient. Modern turbines spray the cooling aerosol from three points around the cutting axis to ensure that the wall which is being cut cannot obstruct the free flow of spray to the cutting tip.

Early turbines required constant lubrication in the form of oil dripped into the air supply line. The exhaust air of such turbines was usually vented out of the back of the handpiece and could be breathed by the surgery staff. Modern handpieces are lubricated with a cleaning-lubricating spray from an aerosol dispenser prior to sterilisation.

Micro-motors

In addition to the turbine, it is necessary to have a slower speed motor to accomplish such tasks as the removal of soft caries, finishing and polishing etc. The speed range of such instruments should run from around 500 rpm up to 100 000 rpm to allow all tasks to be accomplished. High torque at the lower end of the speed range is essential to prevent the instrument from stalling when performing such tasks as the placement of self-threading dentine retention pins.

Micro-motors fall into two categories, air driven and electric driven. The former are cheaper and more robust. The latter are more versatile but more expensive.

Air motors

Two main patterns of air motor are in common use; rotary vane types and swash-plate types. The latter are falling out of fashion rapidly as vane motors improve.

Rotary vane drive air motor

The principle of the rotary vane air motor is illustrated in *Figs 29 and 30*. A central core is offset within a cylinder which it divides up into chambers by means of sliding vanes which seal from the core to the cylinder wall. If compressed air is forced into one of the chambers at the high pressure side, expansion of air within the chamber will drive it towards the low pressure side where the air is exhausted from the system.

Such motors run smoothly and can develop considerable torque. The torque is dependent upon the length and diameter of the motor and the pressure of the drive air.

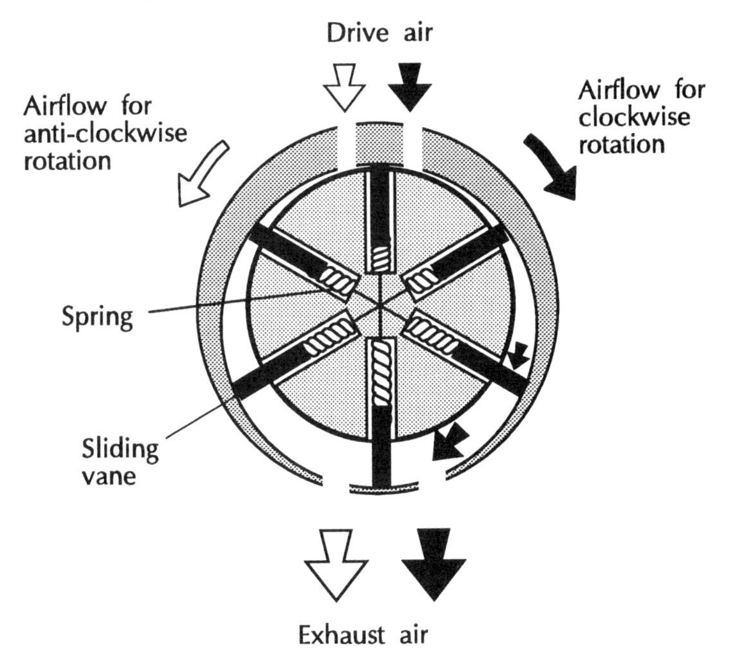

Fig. 29. Principle of the rotary vane air motor.

Rotary vane micro-motors are generally very reliable if correctly maintained although wear on the sealing edges of the vanes can be a problem. One great advantage of these motors is that many of them can be sterilised in an autoclave.

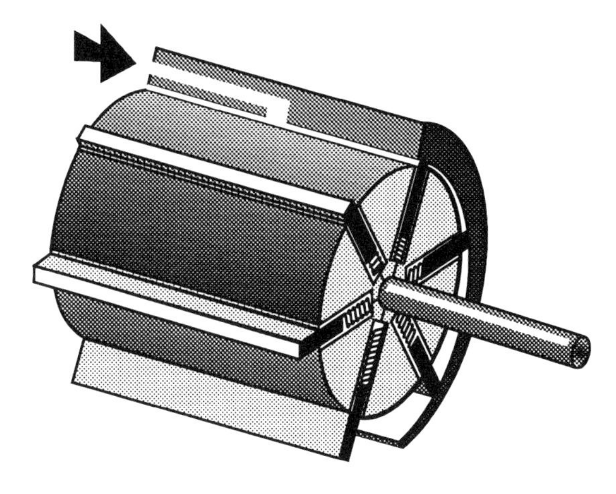

Fig. 30 Cut-away of a rotary vane air motor.

Swash-plate drive air motor

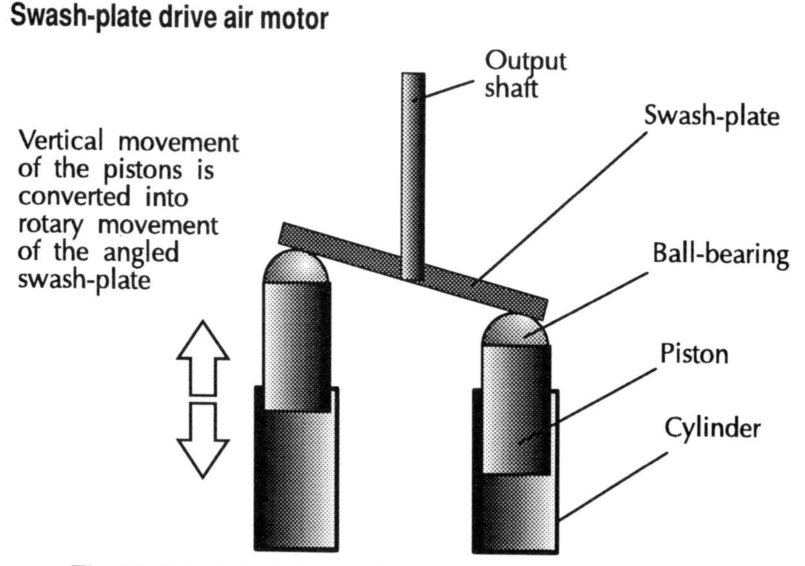

Fig. 31. Principle of the swash-plate micro-motor.

Swash-plate air motors operate by a series of pistons pressing sequentially against a disc which is off-set against its axis of rotation *(Figs. 31 and 32)* As a piston rises it presses against the plate and causes it to rotate. As the piston reaches the end of its travel the next piston in the series takes over and continues turning the disc.

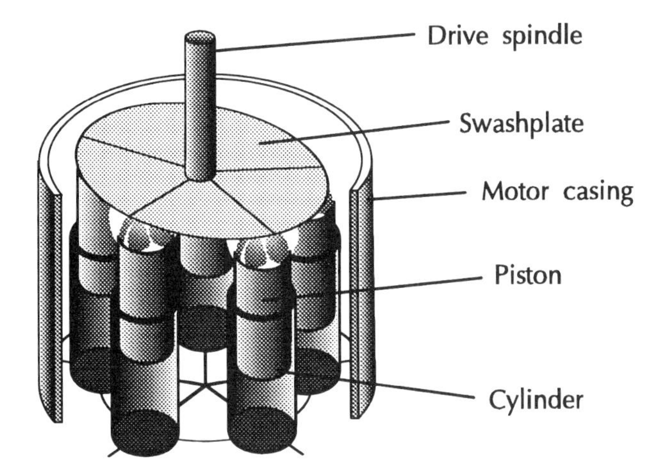

Fig. 32. Swash-plate drive.

The rotation of the disc operates a rotary valve which feeds air to the pistons sequentially.

The swash-plate air motor is not capable of a high speed and is relative noisy in use. It is declining in popularity against the competition of the rotary vane air motor.

Electric micro-motor

Electric micro-motors offer many advantages over air-driven micro-motors. The speed range they can achieve is very much greater and torque control can be very precise. However the overall complexity of the drive system is significantly greater. Electric micro-motors require a supply of cooling air if they are to be run at the higher end of their operating range. An aerosol coolant must be delivered to the cutting bur when higher speeds are in use.

Most electric micro-motors are d.c. motors and are designed with an armature sitting within a permanent magnet assembly *(Fig. 33)*. The performance of d.c. electric motors depends upon the design and power of the field magnets and on the design and number of armature coils. The most powerful d.c. motors utilise lightweight but powerful cobalt–samarium magnets. By varying the distance from the magnets to the rotating armature, the maximum speed of the motor can be altered. This feature is incorporated into some dental micromotors to give two speed ranges, selectable at the motor. The more armature coils, or poles, the smoother and less jerky the operation of the motor. A basic d.c. motor will operate with as few as three poles but most dental micro-motors use either five or seven poles.

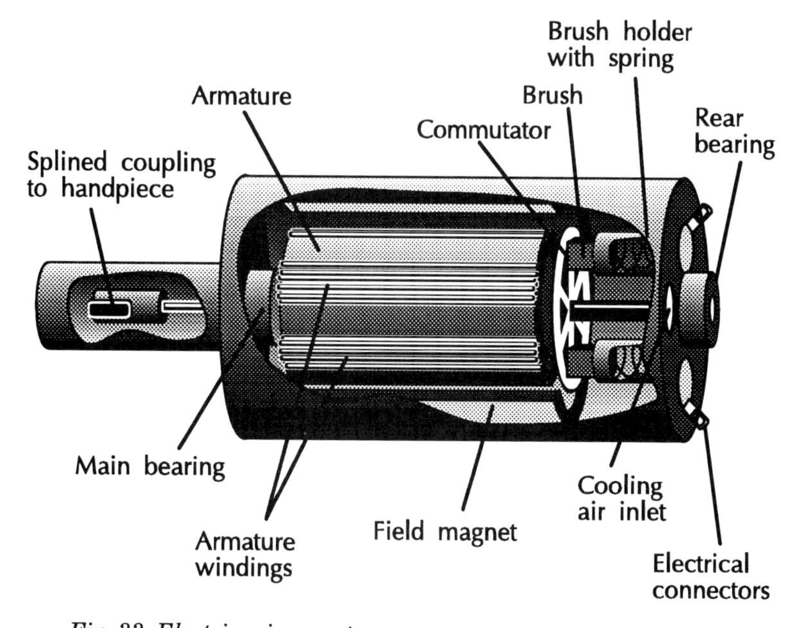

Fig. 33. Electric micro-motor.

Electronic control systems facilitate the operation of electric micro-motors over a very wide speed range whilst maintaining torque. Electronic feedback systems are used which range from simple voltage stabilisers to speed-sensing devices. When a load is put on an electric motor it slows down whilst electrically the current through the motor increases and the voltage drops. Voltage stabiliser circuits will attempt to redress the balance by raising the voltage and in consequence the current until the original supply voltage is reached. This means that more energy is being supplied to the motor so it speeds up to its original speed.

It is not really practical to sterilise the whole of an electric micro-motor and it is better to isolate it from contamination by enshrouding it in a secondary outer casing which can be removed and sterilised between patients. Should sterilisation become necessary then the recommendations of the manufacturers must be considered carefully to avoid damage to the unit. A limited number of electric motors can be autoclaved.

Another type of motor is used sometimes, the electrical induction motor. This uses a contactless armature without a commutator. In place of the permanent magnet which provides the static field the motor uses a series of overlapping field coils which are energised sequentially around the armature. The iron armature contains a number of copper rods within which eddy currents are induced by the field coils. These eddy currents create magnetic fields and these react against the field from the field coils and the armature rotates. Such motors are very effective and quiet but require sophisticated electronic packages to provide the sequential drive currents to the field coils. The speed of the motor is altered by adjusting the rate of sequential switching between the windings of the field coils. Speeds of 40 000 rpm are achieved easily and torque can be maintained under load. Because the only wearing parts are the bearings, the motors are relatively maintenance-free and are very reliable. Like other electric motors air cooling is required.

Couplings

A number of couplings are in use for connecting air turbines and micro-motors to the hoses of the instrument delivery units. Two of the commonest fittings are the two-hole connector and the Mid-West four-hole connector *(Fig. 34)*.

The Borden two-hole connector supplies compressed air through the larger of the two holes and coolant water through the smaller. The Mid-West design has an exhaust tube for removing spent drive air from the turbine and provides spray air and water separately. The ducting of exhaust air leads generally to a quieter handpiece. Many variations of these two main designs exist, for example to pipe in electricity to a micro-motor or supply light to the fibre-optic system of a handpiece. Additionally, some manufacturers use their own unique coupling and in doing so restrict the purchaser to their range of handpieces.

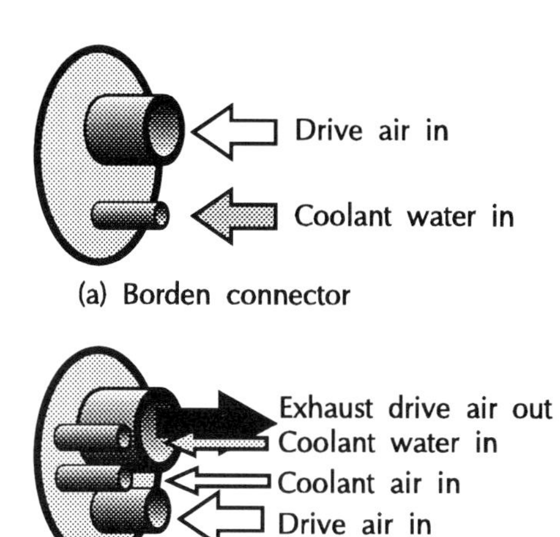

Fig. 34. Handpiece drive connectors:
(a) Borden two-hole; (b) Midwest four-hole.

Many handpieces today offer snap-on connectors. To maintain compatibility between manufacturers it is usual to attach a connector to the supply hose with a conventional Borden or Mid-West coupling and then to snap the handpiece on to this. Snap-on handpieces have become very important since the sterilisation of all handpieces between patients became standard practice. An additional feature of many handpieces today is to allow rotation between the handpiece and the connector so preventing the rubber supply hose from torquing the instrument around whilst it is in use.

Handpieces

Handpieces are the mechanical link between the micro-motor and the cutting bur. Many specialist handpieces exist which drive the instrument in different ways. A handpiece consists of a head and a shank. The head grips the bur whilst the shank connects up to the driving motor *(Fig. 35)*. To allow contra-angulation, gears are an intrinsic component of the system. The gearing in the head of the handpiece turns the drive through 90° *(Fig. 36)*. Both the head and shank can contain gears and in combination alter the speed of rotation and torque.

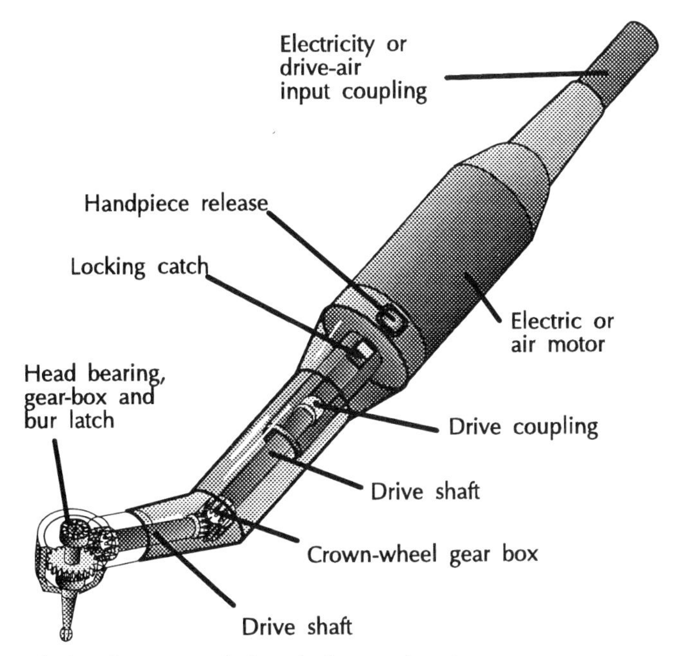

Fig. 35. Contra-angle hand-piece and motor.

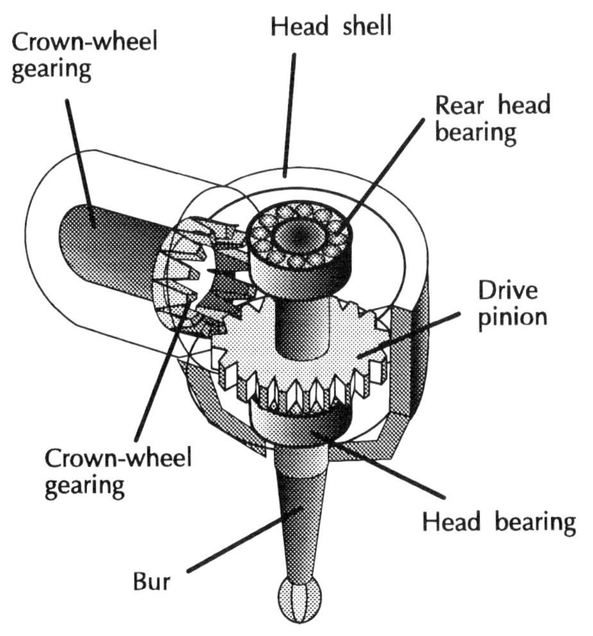

Fig. 36. A speed-reducing head for a contra-angle handpiece.

The E fitting

To allow the interchange of handpieces between motors of different manufacturers, a standardised coupling has been developed. It is referred to as the 'E coupling' *(Fig. 37)*.

The E coupling is an effective and reliable method of transferring the drive to the handpiece. The system uses a simple spring-tensioned dog-clutch which is illustrated in *Fig. 38*. This design ensures a fast and effective snap-on connection without the need to align elements of the system.

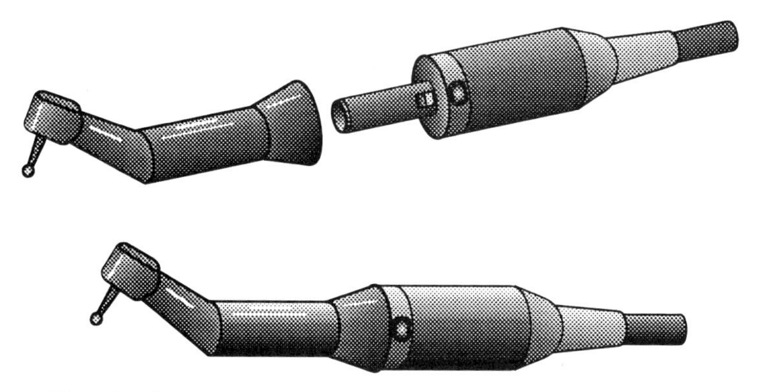

Fig. 37. The standard 'E' fitting.

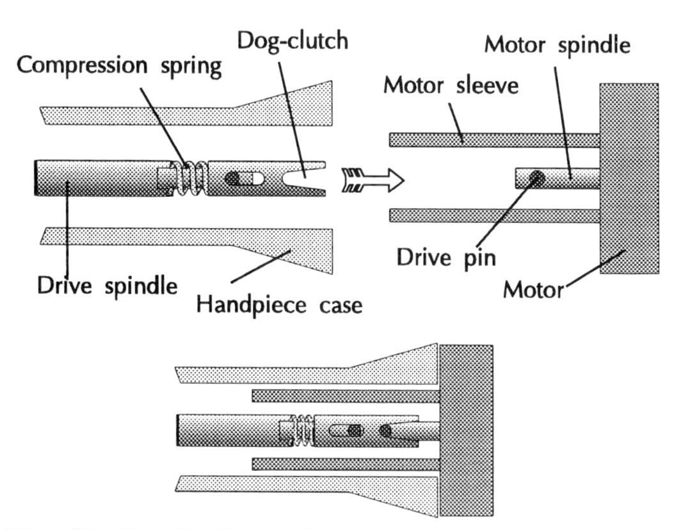

Fig. 38. Dog-clutch coupling mechanism in a E-fitting handpiece.

Coolant spray connecting systems

The earliest E couplings allowed only for transfer of the mechanical drive across the coupling. The coolant spray was delivered via a flexible silicone hose attached between the base of the motor and the head of the handpiece *(Fig. 39)*. This system was later developed to feed the coolant across the coupling within the handpiece *(Fig. 40)*.

Delivery of coolant is not simply a question of squirting water from a tube. To be effective the cooling water must be atomised with a jet of air. Ideally, the air and water are kept separate along two lines within the handpiece and are then delivered from adjacent nozzles in the handpiece head. In this manner, the jet of air breaks up and atomises the jet of water. Simpler systems mix the air and water and then deliver this through a single line to the spray nozzle.

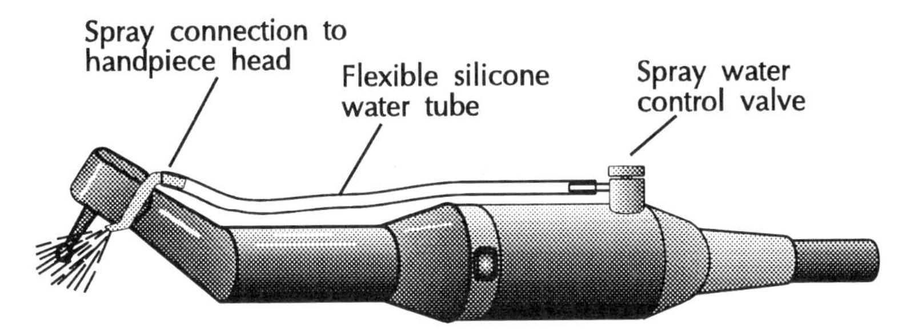

Fig. 39. External water tube between motor and handpiece.

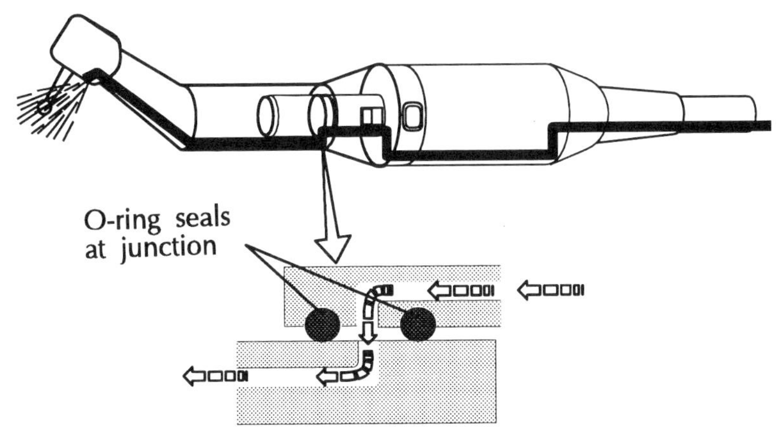

Fig. 40. Internal connection for cooling spray between motor and handpiece.

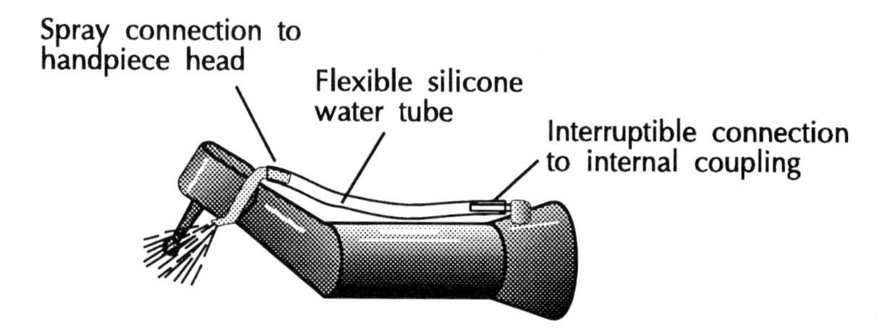

Fig. 41. Externalised spray connection tube allows the use of this handpiece on motors with either internal or external spray connector systems.

The type of handpiece illustrated in *Fig. 41* is particularly useful. It has an E coupling with internal spray connections but then it delivers this spray to the head via an external spray tube. This allows the handpiece to be used routinely with the coolant from the system unit but, when required, an alternative source of coolant can be used. This is necessary when such a handpiece is to be used for surgical procedures such as apicectomies or the removal of third molars. A separate, sterile supply of coolant can be employed.

A further refinement in the E coupling allows fibre-optic lighting to be connected across the joint. Such systems are very sophisticated and increase the cost of the handpieces considerably. Ingenious design allows many of these handpieces to be fitted onto older motors which do not support the advanced features. Similarly, the motors are able to be fitted with older handpieces that require simple mechanical transmission alone.

Control of speed and torque

The simplest handpiece is a straight through, directly linked drive. Both speed and torque can be modified by the incorporation of gear systems. Operative procedures involving rotary instruments can be optimised by the correct selection of handpieces and corresponding gear ratios. Handpieces can incorporate gearing systems of various types but gearing is limited by the need to maintain the drive concentrically through the handpiece and head.

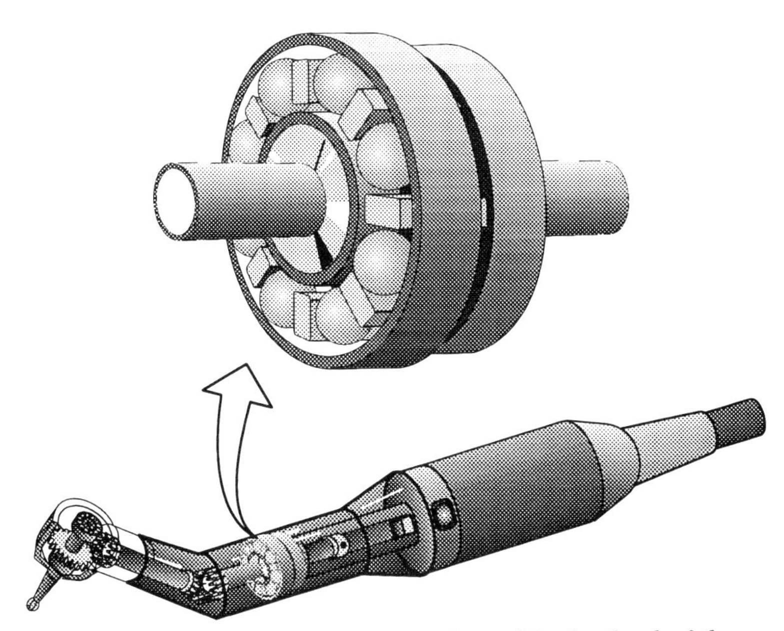

Fig. 42. Epicyclic ball-race gearing located in the shank of the handpiece.

A common method of gearing a handpiece is the use of an epicyclic ball-race gear system. This is usually located in the shank of the handpiece *(Fig. 42)*.

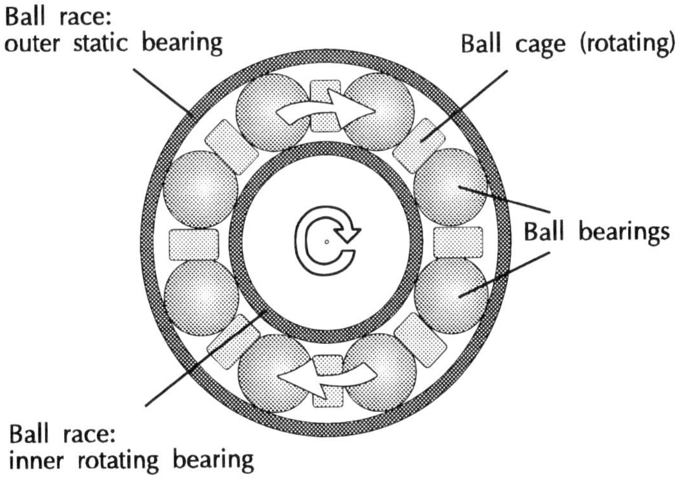

Fig. 43. Principal components of an epicyclic gear box system.

The epicyclic ball-race can be used to either increase or decrease the speed of rotation from the drive spindle depending upon which way around it is mounted.

The basic design is a modification of a ball-race bearing *(Figs 43 and 44)*. If the outer ring of an ordinary bearing is held stationary whilst the inner ring is turned it will be observed that the cage separating the balls turns at a much reduced speed.

This speed reduction is proportional to the relative diameters of the inner and outer rings. In the shank of the handpiece the cage unit is extended and is attached to either the drive shaft or the driven shaft depending on whether a speed reduction or increase is needed.

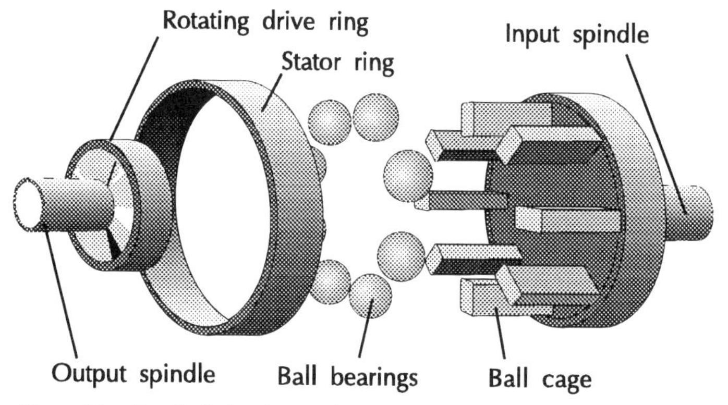

Fig. 44. Exploded view of an epicyclic ball-race gearing system. (Exploded from Fig. 42).

The great advantage of using a ball-race gearing system is that it is very smooth and relatively quiet in operation. Surprisingly high torque can be transmitted without the ball-bearings slipping. Indeed, a modification of this concept has recently been proposed for use in a novel form of automatic gearbox for motor vehicles. Two units can be used serially where larger changes in speed are required.

A further advantage of ball-race gearing units in dental handpieces is that the smooth surfaces of the bearing rings and the ball bearings themselves are relatively easy to clean and lubricate. They resist wear well and function for many years.

Full miniaturised epicyclic gearboxes with toothed gears are now being used in some top range handpieces *(Figs. 45 and 46)*. Provided that these are manufactured from strong alloys and are designed effectively, they can provide excellent and powerful transmission of torque. Such boxes are particularly appropriate for speed increasing handpieces.

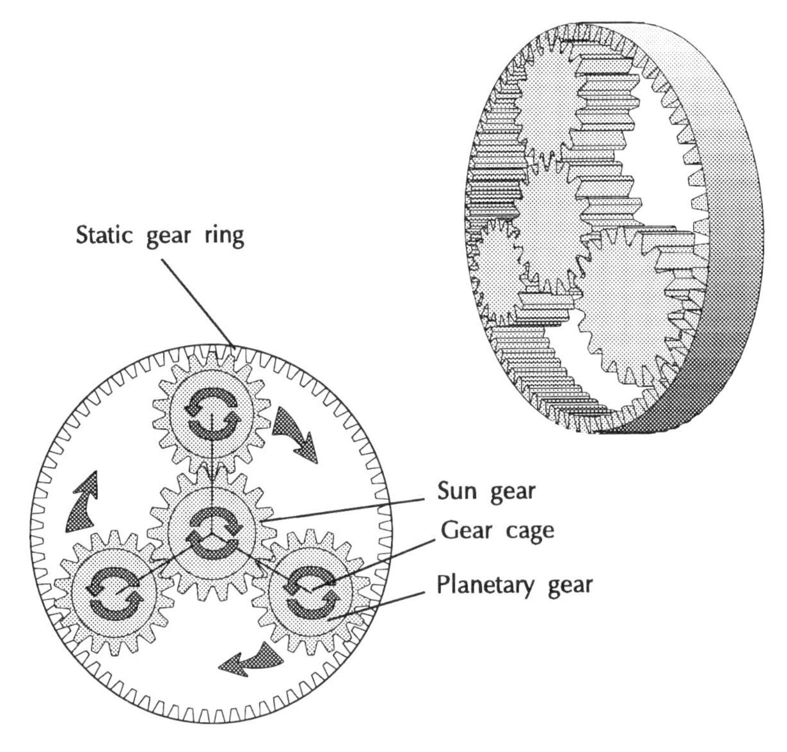

Fig. 45. Epicyclic gearbox using toothed gears.

Reduction handpieces reduce the speed of the drive whilst increasing the torque. These are necessary to drive large diameter instruments such as bristle brushes and rubber cups in prophylaxis heads. Speed increasing handpieces increase the rotational speed at the expense of torque and are designed to drive narrow diameter burs. These handpieces can often be fitted with a friction-grip head to take high-speed burs. With a suitably fast electric micro-motor they can cut tooth tissue as effectively as an air turbine. Electronic control systems can be used to maintain the speed of the motor against the effects of increasing load during cutting. A maintained speed of 200 000 rpm is possible with such a combination *(Fig. 46)*.

Colour-coding

Handpieces are usually colour-coded to indicate the relative gear ratio of each component. Commonly, the head of the handpiece is marked with a coloured dot or ring and the handpiece shank is marked with one or more coloured rings. There is no absolute standard but as general guide blue indicates no change in speed but a straight-through drive. Green indicates speed reduction and red a speed increase. Two or more rings indicate large changes, for example two red rings may indicate a 10:1 increase in speed. The ratio of the head must be multiplied by the ratio of the shank. A green dot 2:1 head in a green banded 2.7:1 shank will reduce the speed of the motor drive to the bur by 5.4:1.

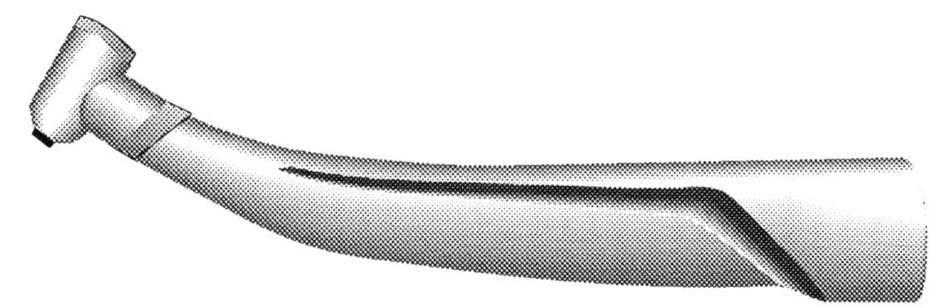

Fig. 46. State-of-the-art handpiece with titanium case, epicyclic speed-increasing gearbox, internal cooling and fibre-optic illumination. (Siemens T1).

Specialist handpieces

Handpieces for endodontics

Endodontic instruments can be driven in a mechanical handpiece provided that a non-rotational movement is used. Endodontic handpieces have been developed which reciprocate, oscillate or both. Some such handpieces require special files whilst some use standard files, gripping the plastic handle in a large chuck.

Handpieces for oral surgery

Oral surgery has led to the development of many types of specialist handpiece, with some designs drifting over to otorhinolaryngology and other specialties in surgery.

Removal of impacted teeth requires fast and efficient removal of bone and sectioning of teeth. Fast rotary vane motors have been developed specifically for such cutting.

Not all operating theatres have clean and dry compressed air supplies. In such theatres alternative systems must be used and it is common to use a cylinder of compressed nitrogen or compressed air to drive dental motors. Electric micro-motors provide a reasonable alternative but may not be acceptable if they cannot be sterilised readily.

Cutting of bone for implant insertion requires cool cutting to avoid local damage due to heat generation. Extremely slow speeds and copious and efficient coolant flow are needed. Additionally, the coolant must be sterile. Special handpieces for implant work are highly geared down to keep the speed low. Special burs are available which are drilled through axially to allow coolant to be piped directly to the cutting edges. Sterile coolant is usually supplied from standard or modified saline drip systems.

CHAPTER 4

Cutting Instruments

Burs and rotary instruments

Several types of instrument are used in rotary handpieces and include burs, twist-drills, abrasive stones and cutting disks. The cutting surface of the instrument may be made of a number of materials such as steel, tungsten carbide or diamond. The specification of a bur is best defined by the ISO standard number 6360. This describes the material of the cutting head, the configuration of the shank, the shape of the cutting head, the grit size and the cutting diameter *(Fig. 50)*.

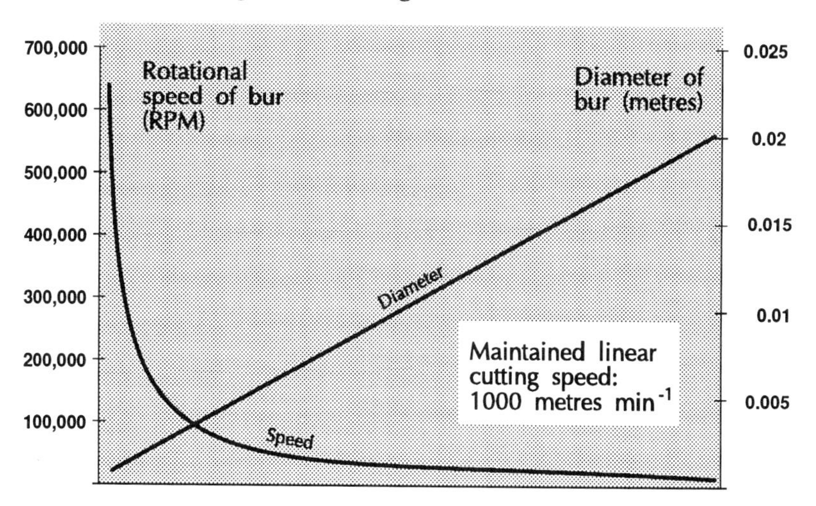

Fig. 47. Relationship between rotary speed and bur diameter to maintain a linear cutting speed of 1000 metres per minute.

Each bur is designed to operate at an optimum speed and is intended for use in a specific handpiece/motor combination. The optimum speed is dependent upon the nature of the cutting material and also the diameter of the instrument. The important parameter is the linear speed of the cutting edge and not the actual rotational speed. A small diameter bur will need to be rotated much faster than a large diameter bur to achieve the same linear blade speed against the substrate being cut *(Fig. 47)*.

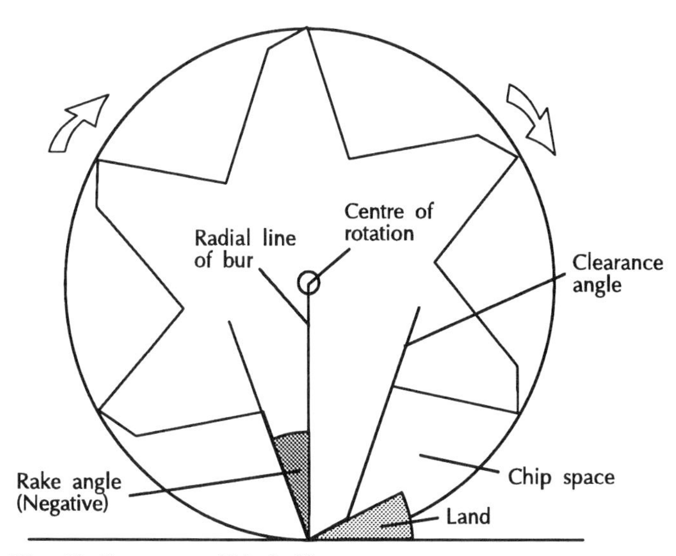

Fig. 48. Geometry of bladed burs.

The basic design of a bladed bur is indicated in *Fig. 48*. Most burs use a negative rake angle although some burs used for cutting soft material such as acrylic occasionally use a positive angle. A range of steel burs for use in a latch-grip contra-angle handpiece is illustrated in *Fig. 49*.

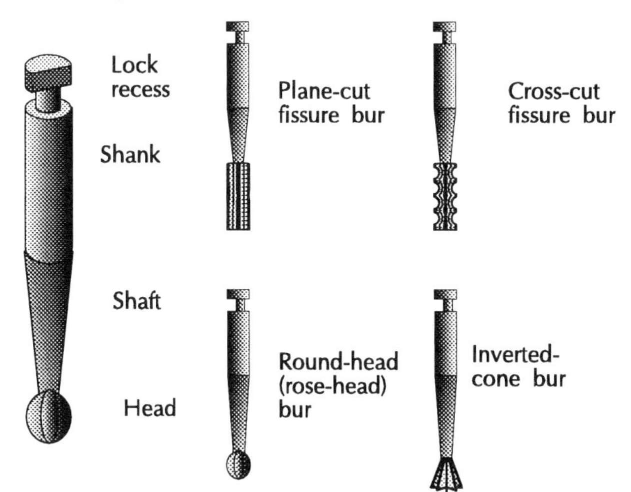

Fig. 49. Range of latch-grip burs.

Bur configuration and specification: ISO 6360

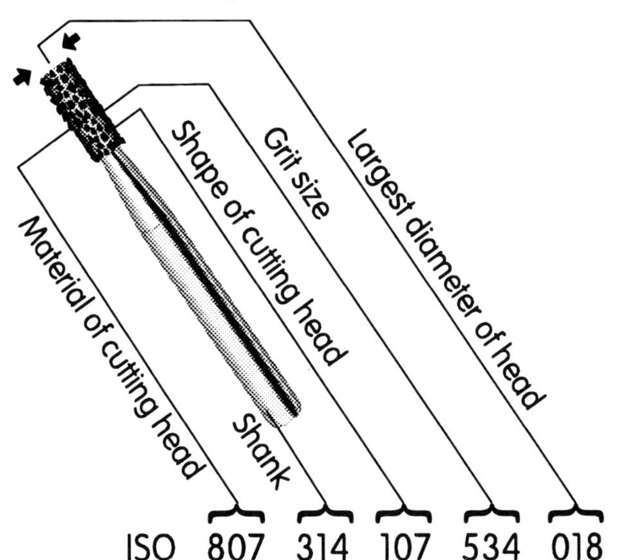

Fig. 50: The ISO 6360 standard numbering system for rotary instruments.

Material

The first three digits describe the material of the cutting edge. The material should be matched up to the material to be cut if effective cutting and optimum bur life are to be achieved.

330: Stainless steel

Steel is the least suitable material for the construction of dental burs. It wears rapidly and corrodes easily in many disinfecting systems. It is, however, cheap and if such burs are regarded as 'single-use, disposable' then it can be effective. Steel is limited to slower speeds. At speeds in excess of 50 000 rpm steel burs deteriorate rapidly.

Stainless steel does not take as good a cutting edge as carbon steel but is more corrosion resistant. It is suitable for sterilisable or disposable burs used in a motor-driven handpiece.

500: Tungsten carbide

Tungsten carbide is an extremely hard material and can be used a very high speeds. It is the material of choice for bladed burs in turbine handpieces. At the high speeds at which this instrument operates, steel burs would be destroyed within a very short period of time. A far harder material is needed to withstand the forces at the cutting edge and tungsten carbide fulfils this need. However, one of the penalties to be paid for hardness is an increase in brittleness. Only the blades of a bur can be made in tungsten carbide, the shank being made of steel. The two components are usually joined by sintering the tungsten carbide blades onto the steel shank.

Tungsten carbide is also very suitable for burs designated for use at lower speeds in motor-driven handpieces when these are to be reused. Because of the extremely fine edge which can be developed on the material, tungsten carbide is also the material of choice for laboratory burs, precision milling burs and acrylic cutters. Instruments made from tungsten carbide are very much more expensive than those in steel but may compensate for this by their much longer service life.

Tungsten carbide is extremely hard but also it is extremely brittle. If it is used inappropriately it will chip or fracture. It is very important to ensure that the correct bur is being used with a particular material. If the rake angle of the bur is not appropriate to the material being cut then damage may occur.

Tungsten carbide burs have a negative rake angle and relatively shallow land *(Fig. 48)* to avoid chipping of the edges. One exception to the blade pattern of tungsten carbide burs is found in the 'Baker-Curson' bur. This bur consists of a tungsten-carbide blank sintered onto the steel shank. No blades are visible macroscopically, but microscopic blades are cut into the surface by stroking the tungsten carbide longitudinally with a diamond stone. This micro-cutting surface produces a very fine surface finish and can be used on most hard materials. The blade pattern can be freshened every time the bur is used by re-cutting the surface with the side of a diamond bur. Because they are resharpened so easily, Baker-Curson burs last for a very long time. Furthermore, the profile of the bur can be customised by running it in an air-turbine and then shaping it with a diamond bur held in the fingers. After the desired shape has been obtained the surface should be resharpened prior to use.

615; 625; 635: Aluminium oxide

These are three specifications of aluminium oxide or 'corundum' used in grinding instruments. They are used mainly in the laboratory but some versions are available for clinical uses such as the bulk reduction of composite restorations. Aluminium oxide (Al_2O_3) approaches the hardness of diamond in terms of useful cutting ability but is considerably cheaper. The best stones are made using a ceramic or vitreous matrix to hold the aluminium oxide particles. They can also be mixed with a strong resin binder and formed into grinding wheels and points but these will be much less durable. One advantage of aluminium oxide points is that they can be custom-shaped by running them against a static diamond wheel or a diamond-coated shaping block.

Aluminium oxide is tougher than silicon carbide but not as hard. It is useful for grinding acrylics, resin matrix composites and metals. Aluminium oxide can react with glass and therefore it is not the best material for grinding porcelain. Silicon carbide is a better choice.

806; 807: Diamond

Diamond-coated burs are the most aggressive rotary cutting instruments available. Whilst diamond will cut almost anything, diamond burs may be less effective in some applications than bladed burs. Grinding can generate considerable heat and if the effect of the bur is to melt the material instead of to cut it then it can become useless soon after application. Diamond grinding surfaces clog up easily and if the debris is not removed but becomes bound up between the diamond particles then the bur loses its cutting efficiency rapidly. The burs require efficient coolant water sprays to clear the chips and keep them running effectively. Frequent cleaning of diamond burs maintains cutting efficiency and minimises wear. Quick cleaning can be done at the chairside with a diamond-cleaning rubber but ultrasonic cleaners with a detergent bath are more efficient.

Diamond-coated burs are available in a wide range of grit mesh or particle size. Coarse grit diamonds are used for removing old restorations and for roughing out tooth preparations. Finer grits are used for finishing margins and finer grits still for the finishing of restorations surfaces.

The durability of a diamond-coated bur depends less on the strength of the diamond particles but rather on the strength of the matrix which is retaining them. A strong and durable matrix which will maintain a tight grip on the diamond particles is the key to a long-lasting bur. Type 806 burs are electro-plated. The diamond particles are held in a layer of metal plated electrically over the surface of the bur. Nickel is used commonly for the plating. Type 807 burs are sintered. Sintering involves melting a metal matrix around the diamond particles and is much stronger than plating.

Shank form

103; 104; 105: Standard handpiece bur

Types 103, 104 and 105 specify a shank diameter of 2.35 mm and a length of 34 mm, 44 mm and 65 mm respectively. 2.35 mm is the usual diameter for a motor-driven bur. The shank of the bur is plain and has no provision for locking into the handpiece. It must be retained in the handpiece by a firm friction chuck. This type of shank is usually reserved for laboratory handpieces but also finds some application in surgical burs which are mounted in straight handpieces.

124: Handpiece bur

Type 124 specifies a shank diameter of 3.0 mm. This is reserved for heavy-duty laboratory burs and requires a special handpiece chuck. It is not a common size.

202; 204; 205; 206: Contra-angle standard

204 specifies a short-shank bur of diameter 2.35 mm with a lock cut for a latch-grip handpiece. The shank lengths are 16 mm (202), 22 mm (204), 26 mm (205) and 34 mm (206). Type 204 is the most common shank configuration for motor-driven handpiece burs for clinical use.

313; 314; 315; 316: Standard friction-grip

Type 314 is the standard bur shank configuration for burs intended for use in the air-turbine. The shank diameter is 1.60 mm and is plain-sided without any locking notches. These burs are held in friction-grip chucks which may be either screw-locked or force-fitting. The other numbers refer to shorter and longer shanks, 16 mm (313), 19 mm (314), 21 mm (315), 25 mm (316).

900: Unmounted grinding points

The 900 designation applies to points which require attachment to a carrying mandrel to enable them to be used in a handpiece. These are mostly instruments for use in the dental laboratory.

Shape of cutting head

001: Round head

The round-head or rose-head instrument is used for general penetration of enamel surfaces and when combined with a bladed metal material is used for the removal of softened and decayed dentine.

010: Inverted cone

In the days of less conservative and more empirical cavity preparation, the inverted cone bur saw much application, but its use in cavity preparation today is very limited.

107: Cylindrical bur

The cylindrical or 'fissure' bur is a general work-horse instrument used for roughing out cavity preparations. Both side-cutting and end-cutting instruments are specified.

168: Conical bur

The 168 pattern has much use in crown and inlay work, being used to develop a line of withdrawal within a cavity design and to determine the taper or cone angle of the preparation.

237: Pear-shaped bur

The main use of a pear-shaped bur is in finishing metal restorations such as dental amalgams. Such burs are usually made of steel or tungsten carbide and have many fine blades to give a smooth and minimal finishing cut.

243: Flame-shaped bur

Flame-shaped burs find use in finishing restorations rather than in cavity preparation. The shape is used to access and refine gingival margins of approximal and gingival cavities. It also helps access some of the finer grooves of the occlusal surface.

260: Bud-shaped bur

Bud-shaped burs are used mainly to reduce the lingual and occlusal surfaces of teeth during tooth preparation for crowns. The shape also has some use in finishing.

284: Torpedo-shaped bur

The torpedo form is used to give a chamfer-edge finish line on tooth preparations. This finish line is required for the margins of cast metal restorations such as gold crowns.

303: Lens-shaped bur

The lens form is rather like a very long and narrow bud-shape bur. Whereas the bud-shape has a rounded end the lens form has a point. It is used mostly for finishing burs.

320: Disks

When used in the mouth, cutting disks require special care to avoid accidents. A hand-held cutting disk can grip into the cut it is making and propel itself along the line of the cut, quite out of control of the operator. Because of this problem a disk-guard handpiece should be employed if cutting disks are to be used intra-orally. A disk guard handpiece is a specially modified handpiece which has a strong metal guard surrounding 270 degrees of the the disk circumference, exposing only a quadrant of the cutting edge.

Smaller diameter disk-shaped burs may be used without a disk guard but care must be taken to ensure that they are used at the correct speed. Many such burs are mounted on a friction-grip (314) pattern shank and can be fitted in the air-turbine handpiece. In many cases this will drive the bur too fast and may damage the handpiece. The upper speed limit of the instrument should be checked. Generally it is much better to use such instruments in speed-increasing handpieces fitted with friction grip heads and attached to an electric micromotor.

The same problems of cutting disks apply in the laboratory and can cause damage to the technician. It is very important to ensure that the disk is chosen correctly for the material to be cut and that it is used at the appropriate speed.

Grit size

494; 504; 514; 524; 534; 544 grit grades

These final figures specify the coarseness of grain of abrasive instruments. 494 is super-fine (15 microns), 504 is extra-fine (30 microns), 514 is fine (50 microns), 524 is medium grit (100–120 microns), 534 is coarse grit (135–140 microns) and 545 is extra-coarse (180 microns). Burs designed for crown and inlay preparations are often available in matched sets of identical shapes but varying grits so that the bulk of tissue can be removed quickly and then the surface finished without losing the shape and form of the preparation.

Hand Instruments

Most hand instruments are fabricated from stainless-steel. Specialised cutting edges can be made from tungsten carbide and then bonded onto a stainless-steel handle by sintering or soldering. Carbon steel produces a very good cutting edge on hand-instruments but is rapidly degraded by corrosion during sterilisation. Carbon and stainless-steel instruments require cutting edges to be reformed regularly by sharpening. Inappropriate sharpening is a fast way to destroy an expensive instrument and great care needs to be taken to avoid this.

Sharpening steel hand instruments

Sharpening, or honing, of steel hand instruments may be accomplished with a hand-held flat stone or using a specially-designed honing machine.

Hand sharpening

A new edge can be put onto a steel instrument quite rapidly and the most important aspect of hand-sharpening is not to overcut the edge or alter its cutting-angle.

The sharpening stone should be lubricated with a few drops of mineral oil. The instrument is aligned carefully and then abraded against the stone using a gentle figure-of-eight movement. When a new edge is formed, the blade is passed longitudinally down the sharpening stone in one or two gentle strokes to refine the edge. The blade should be examined under magnification such as a jeweller's loupe to determine if any swarf is attached to the edge. If swarf is seen then the blade should be inverted and passed gently a short distance over the finest oil-stone surface to remove it.

Machine sharpening

A number of sharpening machines are available. One of the problems of using a powered sharpening stone is that it can remove metal much faster than by hand and can alter critical edge angles if used inappropriately. Machines which use an oscillating stone mimic the action of hand-sharpening and are very effective, especially if combined with a clamp or jig system which enables the instrument to be set and retained at the correct angle to the stone during sharpening.

Sharpening tungsten carbide hand instruments

Tungsten carbide can only be abraded easily by diamonds. The easiest way to re-edge a tungsten carbide instrument is to use a fine diamond-coated disk rotating in a straight handpiece at a speed of 10–50 000 rpm depending upon the diameter of the stone. Spray water cooling should be used. The instrument should be aligned carefully and then brought gently into contact with the rotating surface of the disk until a new edge is formed. Great care is needed because the removal of tungsten carbide can be very fast and if the angle of application of the sharpening stone is incorrect the instrument will be ruined within seconds.

CHAPTER 5

Ultrasonic and Sonic Instrumentation

Ultrasound scaler

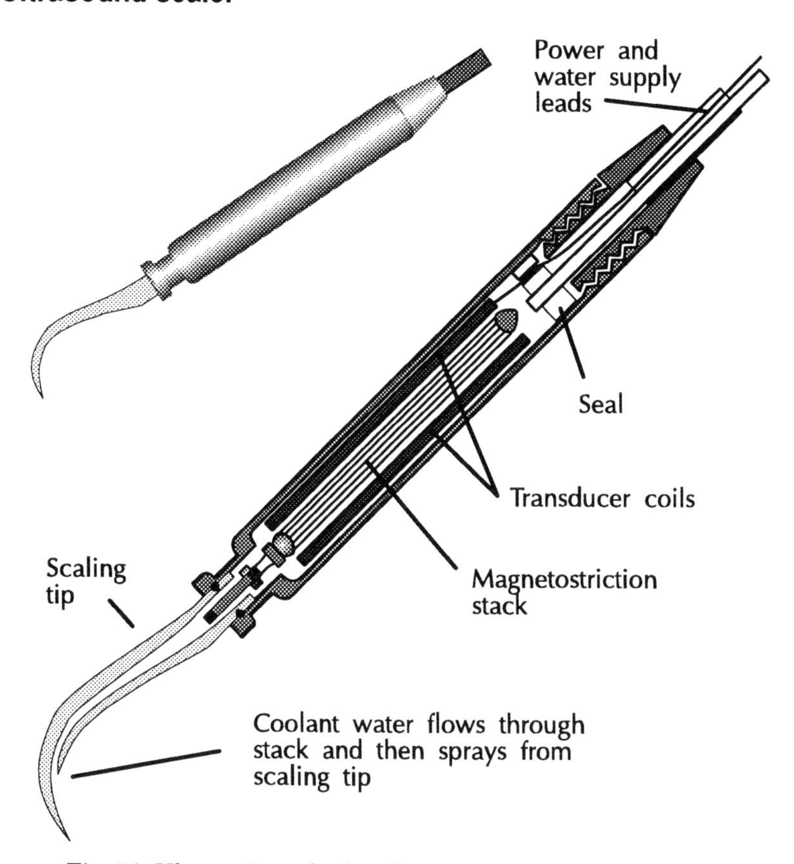

Fig. 51. Ultrasonic scaler handpiece.

The ultrasound scaler *(Fig. 51)* is an instrument in common use in dental practice for the removal of calculus and other deposits from teeth. It has many advantages over hand scaling both in terms of speed and efficiency. Ultrasonic dental scalers utilise three principles in their operation; the direct effect of ultrasound on the calculus, ultrasonic cavitation and acoustic micro-streaming. The direct effect of the vibrating tip disrupts the calculus rapidly and is enhanced by cavitation and micro-streaming. Mechanical scaling effects from the operator tugging at the calculus with the tip of the instrument should not feature in the utilization of the instrument.

Principles of ultrasonic cleaning

Like any other sound wave, ultrasound is the rapid alternation of positive and negative pressure. When in a liquid, the waves of positive pressure increase the local density by compressing the molecules together whilst the negative pressure will decrease the local density by pulling the molecules apart *(Fig. 52)*. This decrease in negative pressure can form cavities in the liquid.

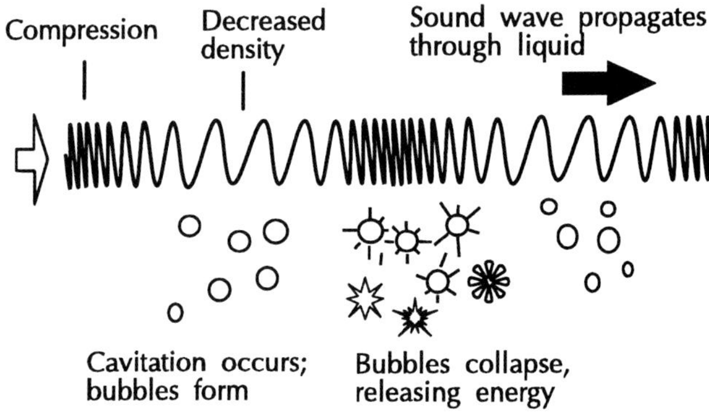

Fig. 52. Cavitation of a liquid by ultrasound.

Cavities, or bubbles, will only form in a pure liquid when the negative pressure is greater than the attractive forces between molecules. In theory, forces greater than 1000 atmospheres would be needed to cause cavitation in pure water. However, water normally contains minute particulate impurities which produce weak points where cavitation can occur under the effects of relatively moderate ultrasound. Once formed, bubbles may grow and recompress in phase with the ultrasound but once they fall out of phase instability occurs rapidly and, driven by the next compression wave, the bubble implodes.

When it is free in a liquid, the bubble remains symmetrically spherical while it collapses. But when implosion occurs next to a solid surface, the dynamics of bubble collapse change significantly *(Fig. 53)*. Jets of liquid are generated which may have velocities of several hundred kilometres per hour as the energy of the bubble is converted into the jet. These may hit the surface with the effect of solid projectiles and erode the surface considerably. It is this energy liberated against surfaces which is exploited in the ultrasonic scaler and the ultrasonic cleaning bath. Surface dirt and debris, which are weaker than the underlying surface, are blasted off rapidly whilst the overall energy of the system is chosen to be less than that necessary to damage tooth enamel or metal surfaces.

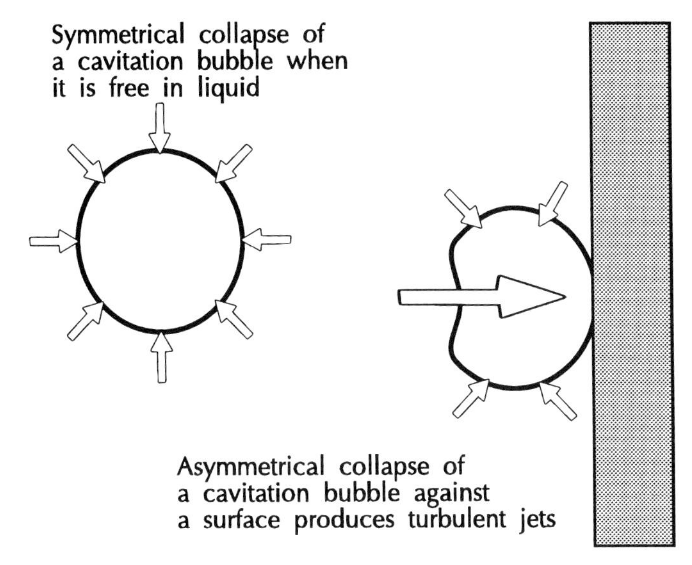

Fig. 53. Formation of energetic jets by ultrasonic cavitation.

Shear forces occur at the tip of the ultrasonic instrument due to acoustic micro-streaming. These forces contribute also to the effective action of the ultrasonic scaler.

As with any other device capable of producing oscillating magnetic fields, care must be taken when using the device on or in proximity to a patient who is fitted with a cardiac pace-maker. Modern, shielded devices should remain unaffected but it is important to consult the patient's physician before treatment.

Ultrasonic scalers create cavitation effects by squirting water over or through a metal scaler tip which is energised by an ultrasonic transducer at a frequency in the order of 25 or 30 kilohertz. Two types of ultrasonic transducer are used commonly, magneto-striction oscillators and piezo-electric crystals.

Magnetostriction transducers

If a piece of iron is placed in a magnetic field it will reduce in overall size by a slight amount *(Fig. 54)*. This effect is known as magnetostriction.

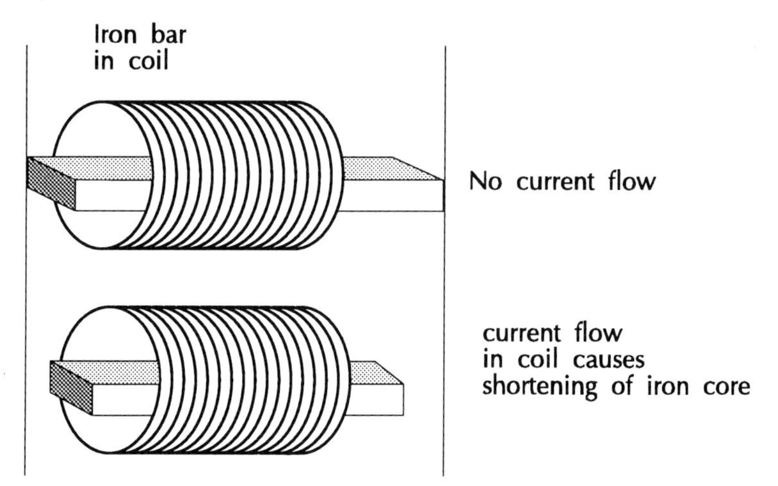

Fig. 54. Magnetostriction.

If the magnetic field is made to alternate then the piece of iron will vibrate at a corresponding rate. This effect is used in ultrasonic scalers to convert the high frequency supply current into ultrasound.

The handpiece of such a scaler contains a coil which surrounds a stack of laminated soft iron strips. When an alternating current is passed through the coil, a magnetic field is produced and the stack vibrates in phase with the current. This is known as a magnetostriction oscillator.

One considerable refinement of this system is to set the length of the stack to correspond precisely with the wavelength of the ultrasound in use. In this way, resonance effects occur and the effective ultrasound energy increases. Early machines were fitted with a tuning control to allow fine adjustment of the frequency to maximise resonance. Modern machines have a feedback control system which adjusts the frequency automatically to optimise the efficiency of the transducer.

When designing such an instrument it is possible to ensure that high stress anti-nodes do not occur at a weak point in the instrument such as a weld or taper. Poorly-designed instruments have been produced which fail to take this into consideration and in consequence showed an unacceptable rate of failure due to instrument fracture. Furthermore, the tip of the instrument can be set at an anti-node in the ultrasound wave so that maximum displacement occurs at the working point. This increases the power and efficiency of the system.

Piezo-electric transducers

When certain crystals are subjected to an electric field they distort. If the field is oscillating then the distortion corresponds to the frequency of the field. This is the principle of the piezo-electric transducer and this effect is used in many everyday devices ranging from microphones through to earpieces. Some ultrasonic scalers use such transducers to produce the ultrasound for their action. They run cooler than the magnetostriction type but are sometimes less effective in use. It is very much more difficult to optimise the design to maximise the resonance effects described for the magnetostriction type.

Sonic scalers

Ultrasonic scalers are relatively expensive and require a package of supply electronics to operate the handpiece. High frequency vibration can be achieved within a mechanical handpiece by means of an unbalanced turbine and this principle is used in sonic scalers. Such a scaler is illustrated in *Fig. 55.* The central core of the handpiece consists of a strong metal armature which is suspended within a three-point bearing. Each bearing element is lined with a thick layer of silicone rubber which allows a limited movement of the armature. The working end of the armature is threaded to retain the scaling tip and is mounted against the interior of the handpiece casing with a strong silicone O-ring. This O-ring limits the movement of the scaler tip. A free-running air turbine is attached to the other end of the armature and is rotated by the drive air to the instrument. The turbine has a hole drilled off-centre to unbalance its rotation. It is this unbalanced rotation which causes the vibrations necessary for the action of the instrument. A water channel in the armature is connected through a flexible silicone hose to a water channel in the body of the handpiece and is used to provide the irrigant spray water to the instrument tip. Insignificant heat is generated by these instruments and the action of the water is limited to irrigation and lubrication at the cutting tip.

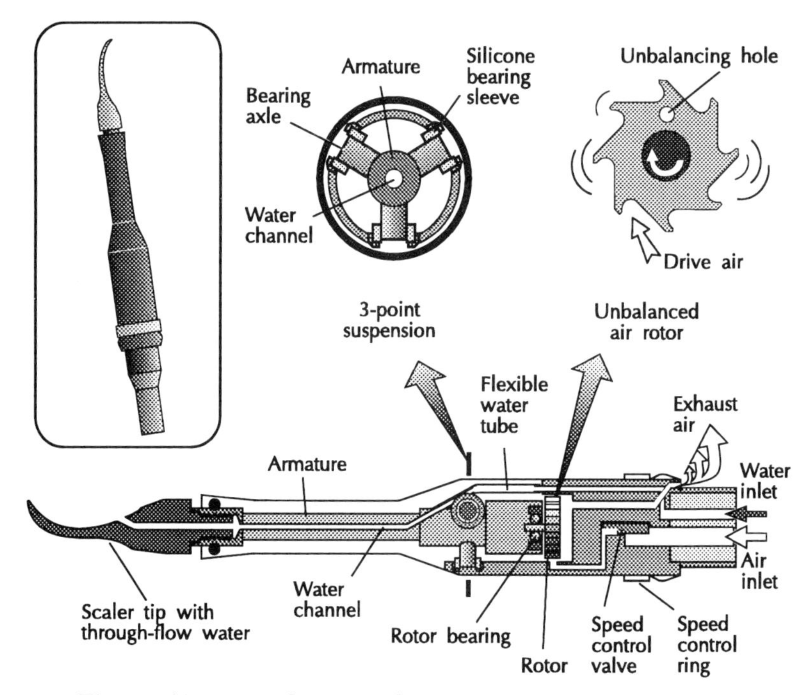

Fig. 55. Air-powered sonic scaler.

When the handpiece is fed with drive air the unbalanced rotor spins and transmits a cyclic vibration through the bearing into the armature. The vibration is transmitted to the scaling tip at the far end of the armature, and is magnified by the lever arm created by the relative distance of the mounting point to the rotor and to the scaler tip. The silicone mountings damp down the vibration and limit its transmission into the hand-held casing.

Ultrasonic cavitation effects do not occur and the scaling effect is purely mechanical. Even so, sonic scalers are effective in the mechanical removal of calculus and have the advantage of simplicity. Often they can be attached to the standard hose of the instrument delivery unit in place of the air turbine or air motor.

Endosonics

Endosonics is the term applied by one manufacturer to the application of ultrasonics to root canal treatment. One of the most important stages of root canal treatment is the biomechanical preparation of the pulp space. Using conventional instruments it is also one of the most tedious. Ultrasonic files increase the speed of shaping the canals, cleanse more thoroughly because of the cavitation effect and relieve the surgeon's fingers of a very tiring procedure. However, tactile sensitivity via the Endosonic instrument is not great and for the best preparation of the apical part of fine canals hand instrumentation is still the method of choice.

The original Endosonic system was a derivative of the ultrasonic scaler and used a magnetostriction transducer (see page 70). The Endosonic file is held by a grub-screw in the head of the ultrasonic transducer *(Fig. 56)*. Irrigant is contained in a reservoir within the system unit and sprays out over the cutting file when the system is in use. Ultrasonic cavitation and streaming effects occur in the solution and assist in the cleansing of the pulp space and in the removal of debris. Various solutions can be employed as irrigants. Sodium hypochlorite is a popular irrigant in root canal treatment but it is corrosive and will destroy the cutting edge of steel instruments quite quickly. This is only a problem if the instrument is to be sterilised and re-used. In sonic and ultrasonic instrumentation this irrigant can cause corrosion of valves and operating parts and should only be used if the manufacturers recommend it specifically. A second supply of water is used to cool the magnetostriction stack.

This through flow of water is sprayed out of the end of the handpiece over the working tip when the unit is being used as an ultrasonic scaler. When it is used as an endodontic instrument the irrigant replaces it and it is ducted back out from the handpiece and into a drain.

The Endosonic device is supplied with two types of file, a fine helical-bladed steel instrument and a diamond-coated instrument. The former is used for the finer preparation of the apical third of the canal structure whilst the diamond file is used for the grosser flaring-back of the coronal two thirds of the canal.

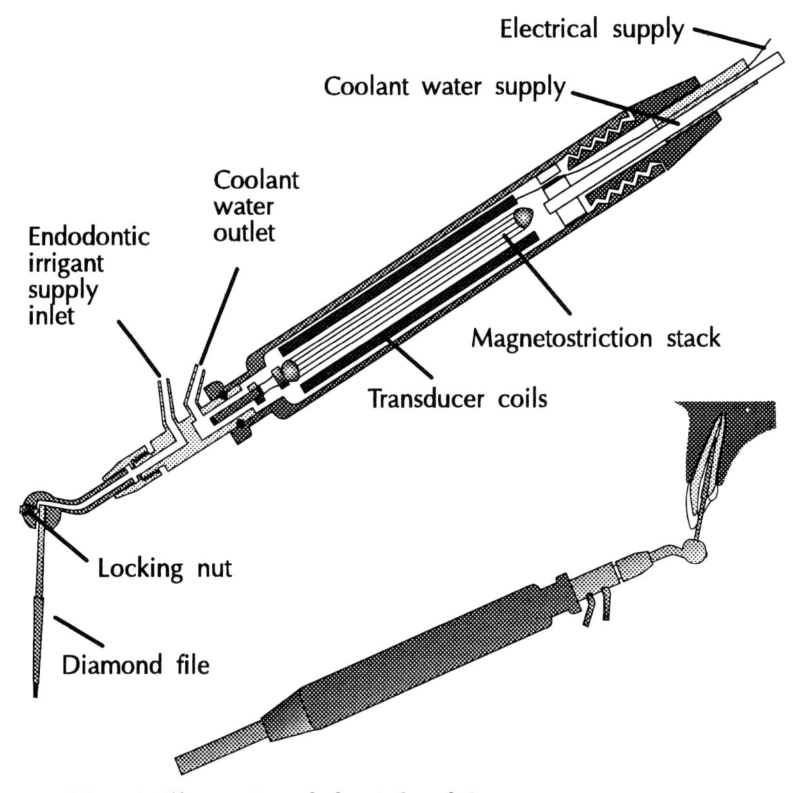

Fig. 56. Ultrasonic endodontic handpiece.

The effects of the ultrasonic canal preparation are mechanical abrasion of the canal walls, ultrasonic acoustic micro-streaming and cavitation which clear debris and thorough flushing of the canal by the copious flow of irrigant.

Like the ultrasonic scaler, sonic systems have been developed as well. These tend to act in a purely mechanical way and do not show the cavitation effects of ultrasound. They are considerably less expensive to purchase than ultrasound devices.

CHAPTER 6

Accessory Devices

Amalgamators (triturators)

Dental amalgam remains a much-used restorative material. It requires energetic mixing of a powdered alloy of silver, tin and copper with liquid mercury. This process is known as 'trituration'. Amalgam alloy powder and mercury may be purchased in bulk or pre-dosed in sealed capsules. The latter method is by far the safest but not the most economic method of handling the materials.

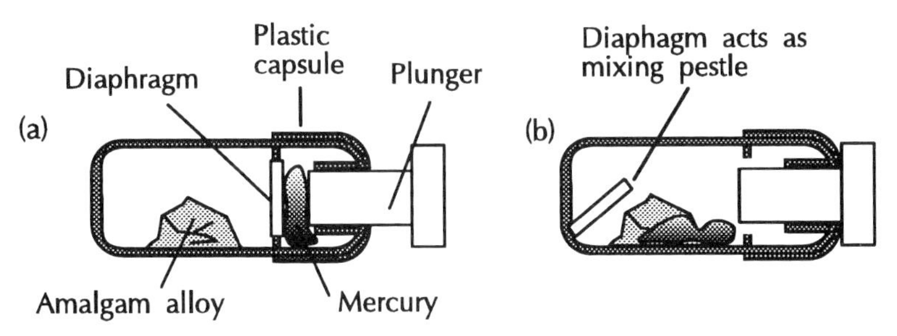

Fig. 57. Amalgam capsules: (a) new capsule; (b) activated and ready for mixing.

Capsules require activation to bring the two components together ready for mixing. This is achieved by breaking two inner compartments into one by telescoping the capsule components together *(Fig. 57)*.

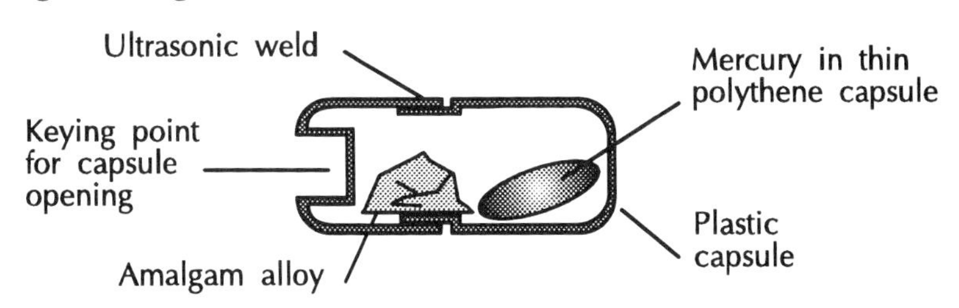

Fig. 58. Self-activating amalgam capsule.

Some capsules are self-activating in that an inner container which holds the mercury ruptures as soon as mixing commences *(Fig. 58)*. Encapsulated amalgam and other encapsulated materials such as glass ionomers are mixed using an amalgamator or triturator. The capsule is placed into a carrying fork which vibrates rapidly and energetically with a cycle length greater than the length of the capsule. This ensures maximum disruption of the contents of the capsule and the most efficient mixing. A timer is fitted to the machine and this can be pre-set for each type of material.

A typical capsule-mixer is shown in *Fig. 59*. An electric motor rotates an eccentric bearing by means of a belt-drive. In its turn the eccentric bearing is connected to a capsule holder.

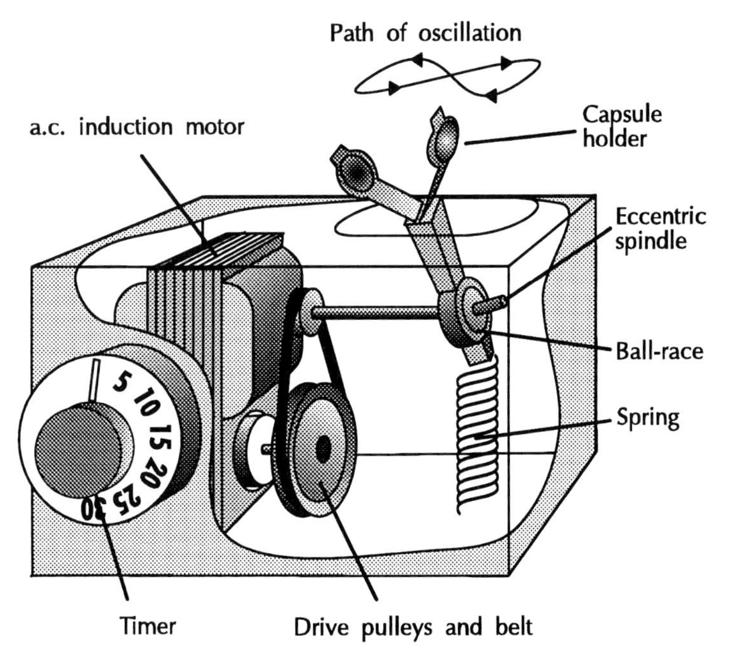

Fig. 59. Operating mechanism of a capsule mixer.

When activated, the capsule is gyrated violently through a figure-of-eight path as shown in the diagram. A typical high-speed mixer operates at around 3000 cycles per minute. The whole inner assembly is suspended on rubber blocks to prevent the unit walking across the bench top as it operates. Many different patterns of capsule mixer have been marketed and the energy of mixing varies enormously. It is vital to check the manufacturer's recommended mixing times against the specific model of mixer in use.

Hopper-feed amalgamators

Powdered amalgam alloy and mercury are cheapest when bought in bulk. To use such products it is necessary to have a device which proportions the alloy and mercury correctly and then mixes it safely without producing excessive mercury vapour. Several types of machine which achieve this are on the market.

The machine contains a hopper for the amalgam alloy powder and another sealed hopper for the mercury. A dosing device at the bottom of each hopper may be activated to tip appropriate quantities of each material down a chute and into the mixing capsule on the front of the machine. The capsule is agitated in much the same way as in the capsule mixer described previously. It is important that the capsule seal is intact and in good condition so that mercury vapour cannot escape while mixing.

The mix of amalgam can be altered by adjusting the ratio of alloy to mercury and by altering the trituration time. Generally, the mix should be kept as dry as possible to limit the amount of mercury used and to optimise the properties of the set amalgam.

Obviously, great care needs to be taken when such machines are being replenished with mercury. Any spillage can be disastrous, raising the mercury vapour concentration in the room to toxic levels if left unattended. The task of replenishment is often left to ancillary personnel and this is a delegation of responsibility which needs to be considered carefully.

Mercury spillages may be tackled by aspirating the mercury up with a large syringe. Every last drop should be chased. Flowers of sulphur should be sprinkled liberally onto the area to absorb any mercury missed by aspiration. Tin-foil can be used to gather up small amounts of mercury because it forms a ready amalgam on contact. Mercury spillage control kits are available commercially. If there is any doubt about the recovery of spilt amalgam then the vapour levels in the room should be checked.

Light-activation units

The first light-activated polymers systems required ultraviolet light to activate them. Nowadays all light-activated materials use intense blue light instead. Usually this light is produced by a tungsten–halogen bulb and filtered with dichroic filters to separate out the required wavelength of blue light at 450 to 500 nm. The light can then be delivered to the restoration in the mouth in a number of ways. Fibre-optic bundles are used in many machines *(Fig. 60).* A fibre-optic bundle consists of many hundreds of fine glass optic fibres *(Fig. 61).* Each fibre is constructed from a fine core of glass surrounded by an envelope of glass of a different refractive index. Light travelling within the core bounces off the walls of the fibre and back in by total internal reflection. The light only leaves the bundle when it reaches the cut end surface of the core. A certain amount of light loss is inevitable along the way due to defects and less than total reflection. Glass is fragile and plastic fibres may be used but these lack the efficiency of all-glass systems.

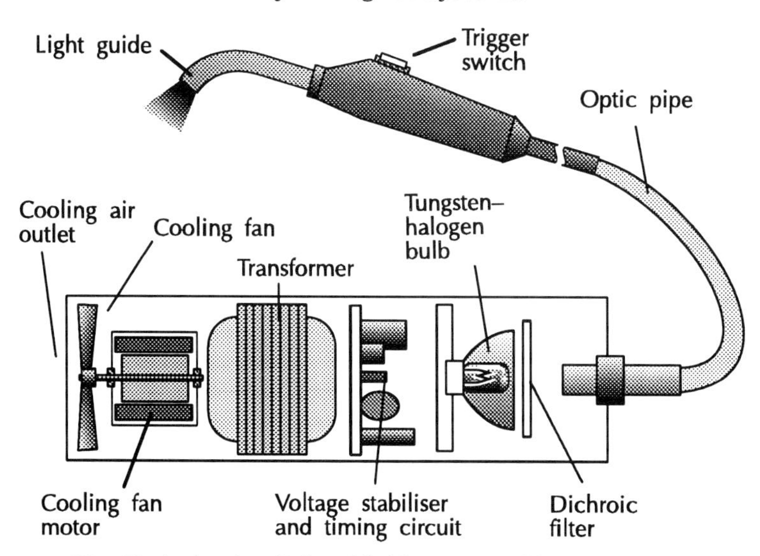

Fig. 60. Activating light with fibre-optic cable.

Such activating units work well and the handpiece is relatively light but the cable is vulnerable to damage. Twisting or curving the cable tightly results in fracture of the light-carrying fibres and the light output is reduced.

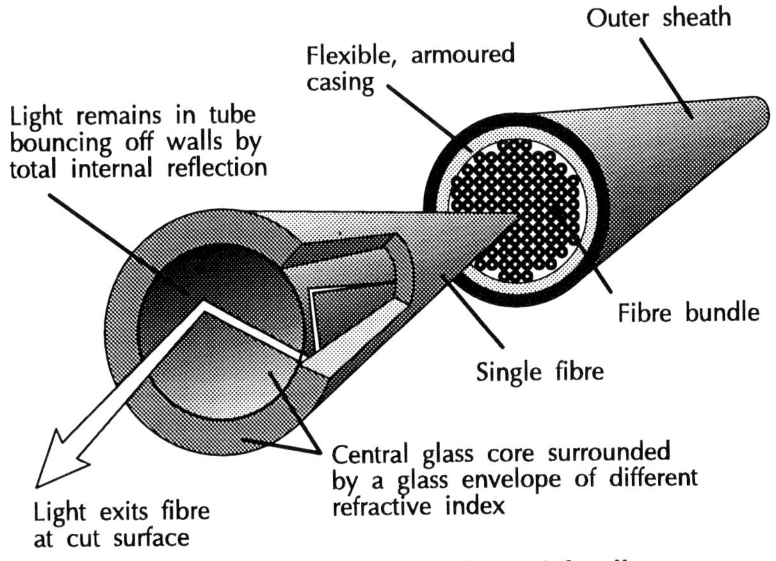

Fig. 61. Light transmission through fibre-optic bundles.

An alternative is to place the tungsten–halogen bulb into a larger handpiece and shine the light via a short rigid light guide into the mouth and onto the surface of the light-activated material. This overcomes the problem of the fragile cable but there is a penalty to be paid in terms of weight and convenience. A fan has to be built into the handpiece to keep it from overheating whilst in use so such machines are generally rather cumbersome and noisy *(Fig. 62)*.

Other factors apart from fracture of the fibre bundle can lead to a reduction in the light output of curing lights. Tungsten–halogen bulbs age quite rapidly and the light output can fall off significantly. Unfortunately they age unpredictably. Variation in the voltage of the mains supply may have a profound effect on the intensity of light output. The more sophisticated units have voltage stabilising circuitry built in to overcome this problem and may be specified to run over a range of supply voltages, for example from 200 to 250 volts to deal with all the supplies of Western Europe.

Monitoring

For the reasons discussed above, the light output of a curing unit may vary considerably. Monitoring is possible using a form of light meter. Several of these are available on the market. They should be used regularly to ensure that the curing lights are operating effectively and that all restorations are being activated right down to the deepest level.

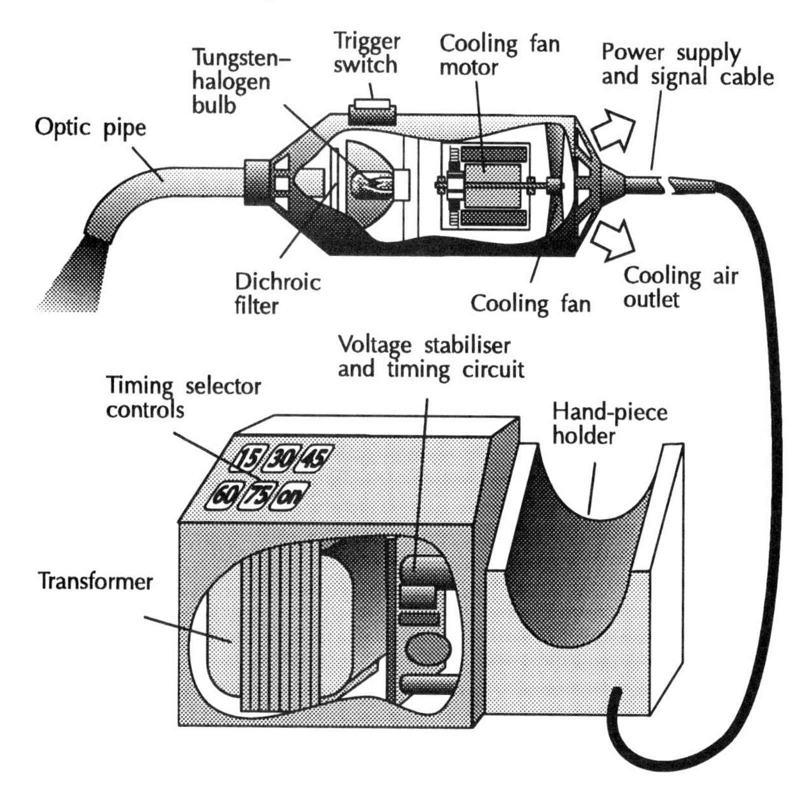

Fig. 62. Activating light with light source in hand-piece.

Safety

The iris of the human eye reduces the size of the pupil in response to bright light so that the retina is protected from damage due to over-exposure. This response is most marked to red light and operates least in blue light. For this reason it is hypothesized that the eye will not protect itself adequately from exposure to the blue light of the activation light and that retinal damage may occur. Filters which remove the blue light are available as spectacles which the operator and assistant wear or as a transparent shield which the assistant holds over the operative site whilst activation is going on. If an activation light is used without eye protection then the operator should ensure that he and his assistant do not stare at the tooth whilst it is being exposed to the light.

Depth of cure

The depth to which a light activation unit can activate the setting reaction of a restorative material depends upon many factors. The depth of the restorative material is important. If the material is placed in a layer greater than the maximum penetration depth of the activation light then the lower aspects of the restoration will never set.

Similarly, the distance from the optic of the activating light to the restorative will determine the intensity of light available in the restorative material. The output of the light decreases according to the inverse square law so doubling the distance from the glass bundle will quarter the light intensity.

The opacity of the restorative material is important. Some manufacturers specify very different activation times depending upon the shade of the material in use. A light, translucent colour will allow far greater penetration depth than a darker, more opaque colour.

The relative sensitivity of the activation chemistry can be altered, but if it is made over-sensitive then the material can start to set under the ordinary operating light before it is placed fully.

The intensity and wavelength of the light are determined by the bulb and the filters as described above and affect the efficacy of the activation system profoundly.

Endodontic filling devices

The objective of root canal treatment is to seal off the root of the tooth at the apical constriction. Many sealant systems have been tried over the years but the one which remains the de facto standard is lateral condensation with gutta percha. Points of gutta percha are coated with a sealant paste and are inserted into the root canal. A pointed instrument known as a lateral condenser is forced alongside the gutta percha and used to deform it against the walls of the prepared root canal, forcing sealer into the fine details of the pulp space. Further gutta percha points are added into the space created by the lateral condenser and then the condensation procedure is repeated until the pulp space is obturated fully. Various devices have been invented to facilitate this process. Several systems use a hot-melt gutta-percha gun to provide a flowing paste of molten gutta percha which can be injected directly into the pulp space. The problem with such a system is that it is very difficult to constrain the pressure-injected gutta percha to the root canal unless a distinct and impenetrable apical stop has been achieved during biomechanical preparation.

One device which facilitates lateral condensation is the 'EndoTech'. This is a simple but effective device which is little more than a lateral condenser heated by an electric element and powered by a rechargeable nickel–cadmium battery. However, it is capable of melting gutta percha well and excellent root fillings can be obtained rapidly and effectively if the device is used correctly. Because it uses a standard lateral condensation technique, it is easier to establish the apical limit of the gutta percha than with the pressure-injection systems.

Bleaching units

Some discoloured teeth may be treated in a conservative manner by removing the stain by bleaching. Teeth stain for a number of reasons including drug side-effects and breakdown of dead pulps. Bleaching may be attempted in either vital or non-vital teeth. In the former case the bleaching agents are applied to the outer surface of the tooth, in the latter case they are applied to the inner aspect through the access cavity of root canal treatment. Bleaching of teeth is usually accomplished by the application of strong hydrogen peroxide to the dentine together with heat to break down the peroxide with the release of nascent oxygen. Direct heat or strong light with a large infra-red component are both effective. Small quartz–halogen lights are available in purpose-built units. These have collimating filters and lenses to focus the light onto the tooth to be bleached.

Heat alone can be provided by an instrument heated by holding it in a gas flame or heated independently by electricity.

Airbrasive polishers

Airbrasive polishers use a principle similar to that of the sandblaster in that they fire a jet of water with abrasive particles against the surface of the tooth. Various abrasive agents have been used. The most popular being a mix of sodium bicarbonate and calcium phosphate.

With a system which has a powerful effect with limited controllability, care has to be taken that its effects are not misdirected. It is important not to blast the abrasive forcefully into periodontal pockets or against damaged tissue.

The unit requires compressed air, water and electical supplies for operation. If it is to be plumbed in, it would be prudent to add isolating valves which could be switched off every night. Such a system is sensible for this or any related surgery add-in which is capable of switching its own water supplies.

Intra-oral sand-blasters

A small intra-oral sand-blaster, marketed as the 'Micro-Etch', has recently become available and is relatively low cost. This is a pencil-sized device which is propelled by compressed air from the dental unit. A small hopper on the top can be charged with fine particle grit. The device is used to produce a micro-mechanically roughened surface on ceramics, metals and composites either intra-orally or at the chairside. Such treated surfaces are more amenable to adhesion.

CHAPTER 7

Thermal Surgery

Lasers

LASER is an acronym of Light Amplification by the Stimulated Emission of Radiation. This title describes the method by which a laser operates. A small amount of light is input into the system and is amplified to a greater intensity before it is re-emitted.

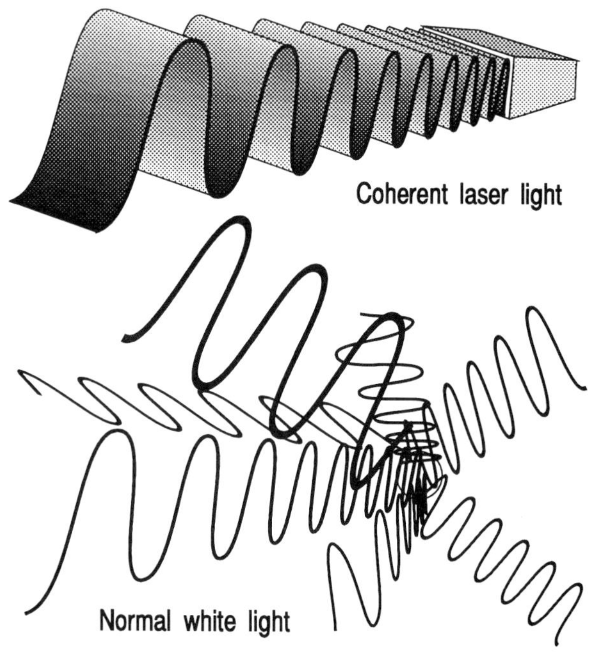

Fig. 63. Laser light is coherent; it is of a single wavelength and the light waves are orientated in one plane. By contrast, white light consists of light at many different frequencies, amplitudes and orientations.

Laser light has a number of distinct characteristics; it is monochromatic, polarised and unidirectional *(Figs. 63 and 64)*. It can be of extremely high intensity although not all applications demand this.

How lasers work

In normal conditions, atoms arrange themselves so that there are more in lower energy states than in higher energy states. In this form, the system is capable of absorbing energy. Heating simply increases the energy of the whole system, the ratio of atoms in a high energy state to those in lower ones remaining the same. However under certain conditions this ratio may be changed and a state known as 'population inversion' occurs. This change is brought about by exciting the atoms selectively to allow those in the higher energy states to keep their energy for a longer period than usual.

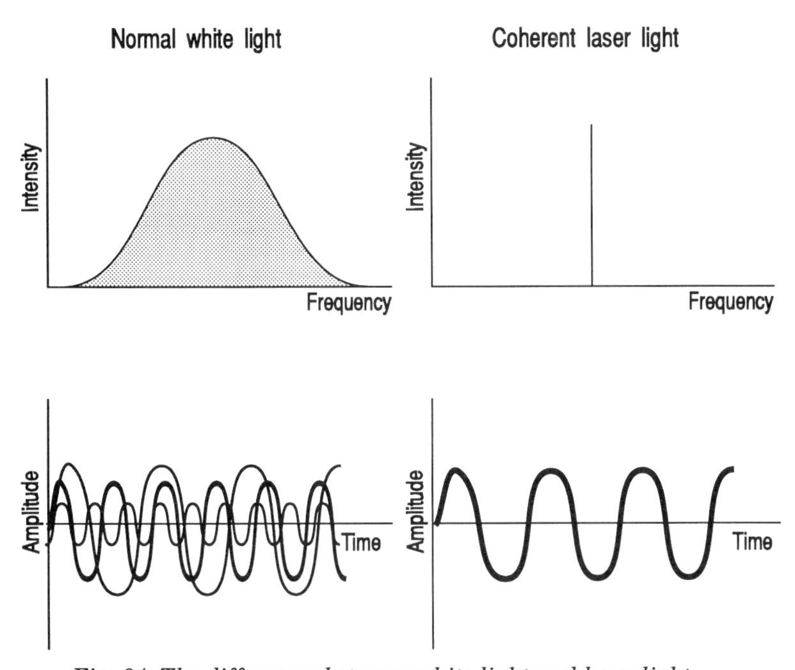

Fig. 64. The differences between white light and laser light.

This excitation energy can be gained from light from other sources, by passing electrical currents through gases or semi-conductors or by chemical reactions *(Fig. 65)*.

If a photon of light hits an excited atom then an unstable state is induced and the atom returns to the lower energy state, releasing the energy as the original photon plus a stimulated one with the same properties *(Fig. 66)*. These two photons then hit other excited atoms and cause a propagation, or amplification, effect. This cascade effect continues until the energy states of the excited atoms are returned to normal. Such a system would produce a flash of laser energy. If the system continues to be excited, or pumped, then the laser effect may produce a constant beam.

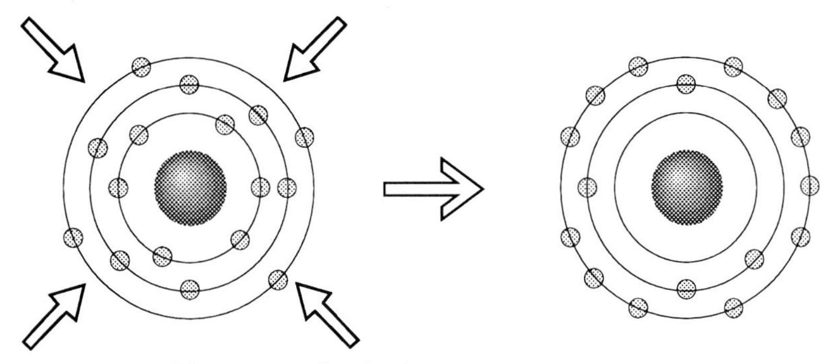

Fig. 65. The process of excitation.

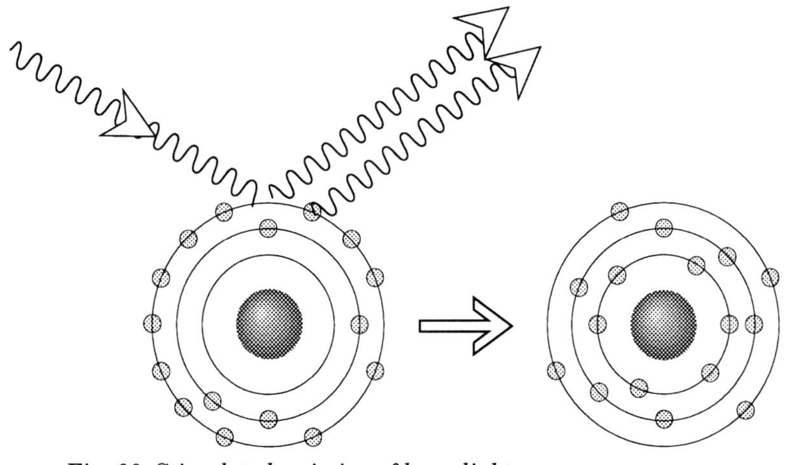

Fig. 66. Stimulated emission of laser light.

Various systems are used to produce laser energy. Small gas-filled tubes are used in the helium neon laser. Ruby crystals, ytrium–aluminium–garnet (YAG) and other solid crystal materials are used in some machines whilst the most powerful use flowing carbon-dioxide gas which is excited electrically. Each type has specific characteristics of wavelength and intensity which may be applied in individual applications.

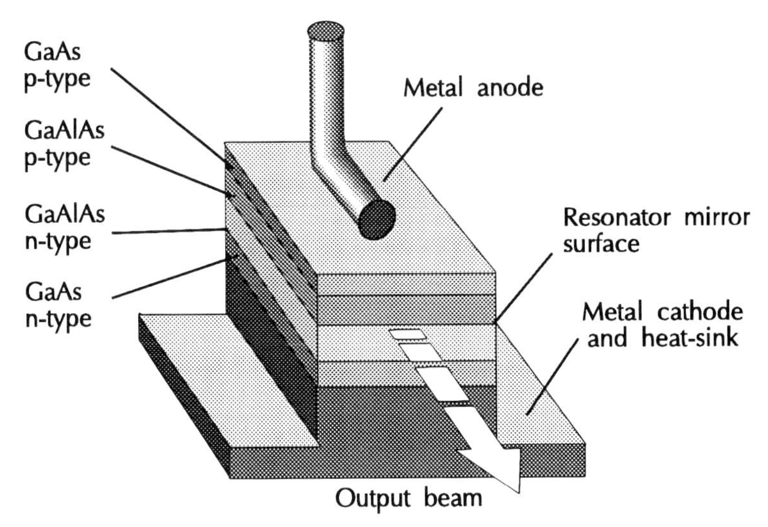

Fig. 67. Heterogenous junction semi-conductor laser.

A semiconductor laser is illustrated in *Fig. 67*. Early semiconductor lasers required cooling systems and could only work in short bursts. A typical material for the laser semiconductor is gallium arsenide. Modern heterogenous junction semi-conductor lasers can work continuously at room temperature without the need for external cooling.

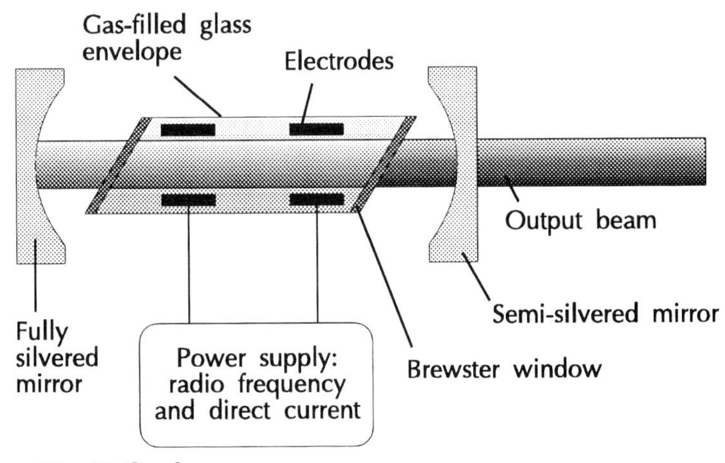

Fig. 68. Gas laser.

A simple gas laser is depicted in *Fig. 68*. The gas is contained in a glass tube which has glass windows at each end specially angled to minimise reflection. These are known as Brewster windows. The gas is stimulated or pumped by a source of radio-frequency and direct current. Spherical mirrors reflect the laser energy across the tube but one of the mirrors is semi-silvered to allow the output beam to pass. The frequency of the output beam will depend upon the particular composition of gases used in the tube. Helium–neon mixes produce an intense red. Carbon dioxide is used to produce an infra-red beam and is the laser of choice for high power applications such as laser surgery.

The prime use of lasers in dentistry lies in oral surgery where they are used to deal surgically with oral malignancies. A high energy laser beam allows pressure-free cutting to cut away the tumour with a minimised risk of seeding the tumour to other sites. The main type of laser used for this purpose is the carbon dioxide laser. This produces a beam of adequate energy for vaporising tissue.

Lasers are not very good at cutting teeth. Enamel and dentine are relatively transparent at most wavelengths from infra-red to ultraviolet. This means that little laser energy is absorbed and so vaporisation of the tissue is limited. The transmitted energy may be absorbed well at the dental pulp and cause considerable damage. Lasers are marketed commercially for use in the removal of caries. Extremely short, high intensity pulses of light are fired at the carious lesion. These are effective at the surface of the lesion and erode it away. However, the residual cavity has a shape with little structural validity and may not be conducive to restoration with contemporary materials.

Experimentally, fissures in the occlusal surfaces of teeth have been sealed with laser beams. Indeed it is possible to 'weld' them closed by fusing hydroxyapatite powder into the fissure system. This has a number of disadvantages which are likely to prevent its widespread use. Firstly, the laser beam used to fuse the hydroxyapatite is quite capable of causing vast tissue damage if fired inappropriately and presents an ocular hazard for the patient and the dental personnel. Secondly, an hydroxyapatite sealant can develop dental caries!

Lasers can be used investigatively and have been used to determine the flow of blood through the dental pulp in the living tooth. This is known as laser doppler flowmetry. The technique has been applied experimentally in the determination of pulp vitality.

So-called 'soft lasers' are the subject of many claims of dubious reliability. Such devices are marketed with an extraordinary range of applications. It has been claimed that the devices reduce the inflammation of periodontal disease, promote healing, encourage haemostasis, accelerate the healing of extraction sockets, etc. Most of these devices are extremely low-powered sources of laser energy. Sunshine would contain light energy of the same wavelength and at far greater intensity than these machines put out. Generally these devices should be treated with appropriate caution and claims of efficacy examined with close scientific scrutiny before purchase is considered.

Diathermy

Diathermy is the localised heating of tissue by a radio-wave. At low powers this form of heating is used by physiotherapists and is known sometimes as 'deep heat' treatment. When a high power radio wave is delivered directly to a small area of tissue the heat is concentrated locally and may be used to disrupt the tissue. This technique is used in surgical diathermy systems, or electrosurgery units.

Dental diathermy units are usually limited to about 50 watts output and operate at a frequency from 1 to 30 MHz. Most units operate at around 2 MHz.

Diathermy units are very useful in dentistry because they provide relatively pressure-free cutting of friable tissue. They also produce some degree of haemostasis around the wound.

The nature of the cut is dependent upon the wave-form and intensity of the electromagnetic radiation which is produced by the diathermy unit. The terms 'section' and 'fulguration' are sometimes applied to the techniques used. If the radio-wave is of a stable frequency and intensity and has a smooth sinusoidal form then clean cutting, or sectioning, results. Sectioning is accomplished with a smooth stable sine wave. If the radio-wave is spiky and of rapidly varying wavelength and intensity then a different effect on the tissues is found. Localised heating tends to 'cook' the tissues and this effect is used to produce haemostasis. A rougher, spikier wave-form again produces another effect. Sparks will jump between the electrode and the tissue before the electrode comes into contact. This arc is used to 'plane' the tissues and the effect is known as fulguration. It has a rather limited use but has found favour in the removal of soft tissue lesions such as those of denture stomatitis.

As with any other device capable of radiating oscillating magnetic fields, care must be taken when using the device on or in proximity to a patient who is fitted with a cardiac pace-maker. Modern, shielded devices should remain unaffected but it is important to consult the patient's physician before treatment.

Cryosurgery

Cryosurgery is the use of extreme cold in treating soft tissue lesions. Tissue can be destroyed by freezing and thawing, provided that a sufficient drop in temperature occurs, and such cellular death is the object of cryosurgery.

Cryosurgery is best accomplished by putting the tissue through a number of cycles of rapid deep freezing, maintenance of the ice-ball for a period of minutes followed by slow thawing. The formation of intra-cellular ice crystals, electrolyte shifts and ischaemic infarction caused by micro-thombi in damaged supply vessels all contribute to cell death within the ice-ball. Various tissues respond to freezing in different ways. Epithelium is destroyed rapidly whilst fibroblasts are more resistant.

Cryosurgery can be carried out with or without anaesthesia. The healing phase is usually uncomplicated and infection is rarely a problem. Post-operative pain is minimal compared with other modes of treatment but there is considerable oedema and swelling. Cryosurgery has particular use in the treatment of tumours and premalignant lesions but also finds use in the treatment of haemangiomata, granulomata and other benign conditions. One of the major advantages of cryosurgery in the treatment of malignancies is that, in theory, all the malignant cells are trapped in the ice-ball and minimal disturbance of the tumour occurs.

The extreme cold can be produced in several ways. The most basic being to dip cotton wool into liquid nitrogen and apply this to the tissue. More sophisticated devices exploit the Joule–Thompson effect *(Fig. 69)*.

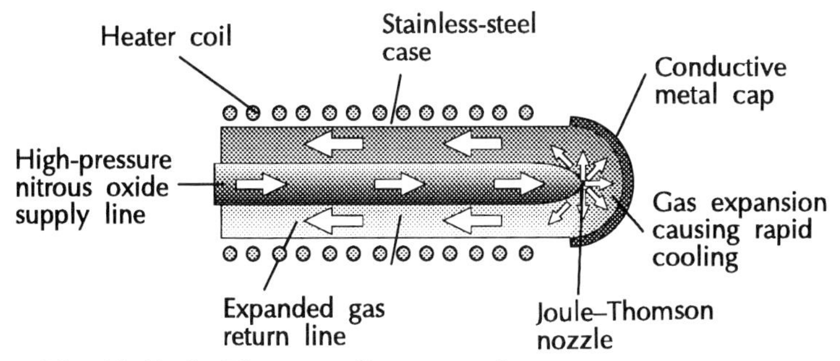

Fig. 69. Joule–Thomson effect cryoprobe.

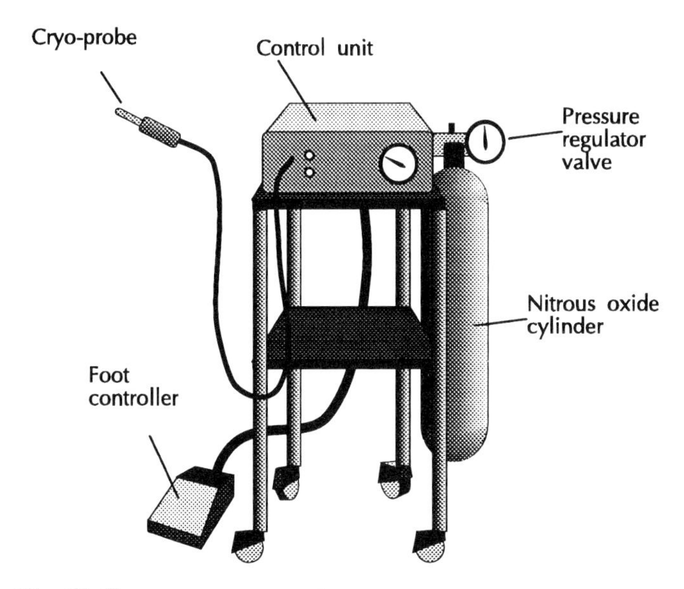

Fig. 70. Cryosurgery apparatus.

This effect is the rapid cooling which occurs when a high-pressure gas expands through a narrow orifice into an area of low pressure. The expansion of gas absorbs heat energy and objects in contact with the gas are forced to give up heat. Such apparatus can reduce temperatures to –70^{0}C rapidly. Nitrous oxide cylinders are a convenient source of gas at high pressure *(Fig. 70)*. The gas pressure at the nozzle is usually in the order of 5MPa.

Superior versions utilise electrical heating coils to release the cryoprobe from the icy tissue surface. The heaters are energised automatically when the foot control is released.

A further enhancement is the use of electrical thermo-couples inserted into the tissues to monitor the temperature fall inside and peripheral to the ice-ball. This helps to ensure that the cryosurgery is effective thoughout the treatment region. This is vital when the technique is being used for the treatment of tumours.

CHAPTER 8

Computer-Assisted Restorative Dentistry

Computer-aided design and manufacture

Computer-Aided Design and Computer-Aided Manufacture (CAD/CAM) systems have been used for many years in various industries, notably the automotive industry, but are now finding applications development in dentistry.

CAD is the use of computer systems in the design and development of a product. The computer is used as an extended drawing board, allowing three-dimensional modelling and design. Mathematical modelling of the structure allows some aspects of its performance to be assessed before it ever leaves the drawing board.

CAM is the use of a computer system to operate machine tools. This allows the shaping of materials to form structures and devices. The computers controlling the machine tools can operate from instructions set up by the computer-aided design system. In this way a complete integrated system is set up. The object to be made is designed on a computer screen and then the design is implemented by the computer.

Restorative dentistry has been restricted by the range of fabrication technologies available. Direct placement restorations are limited to the alloying of dental amalgam, acid–base reactions or the polymerisation of resins. Laboratory-fabricated restorations are limited to lost-wax casting, porcelain sintering or resin polymerisation. This restricts the range of materials which can be used. CAD/CAM systems open up a range of new material systems by providing a new method for the control of shape.

The major limiting factor in applying CAD/CAM technology to dental restorations is that the preparation of the tooth is the prime factor which determines the shape of the final restoration. This means that some method of scanning the tooth preparation accurately needs to be employed. Various methods of achieving this are being tried. The first system which became available commercially was developed in Zurich by Werner Mörmann and marketed by Siemens of Germany. This is the 'CEREC' system *(Fig. 71)*. At the time of writing this system is the only commercially-available chair-side dental CAD/CAM system on the market. Its value and effectiveness have been demonstrated in many scientific studies and over 1000 machines are in clinical use.

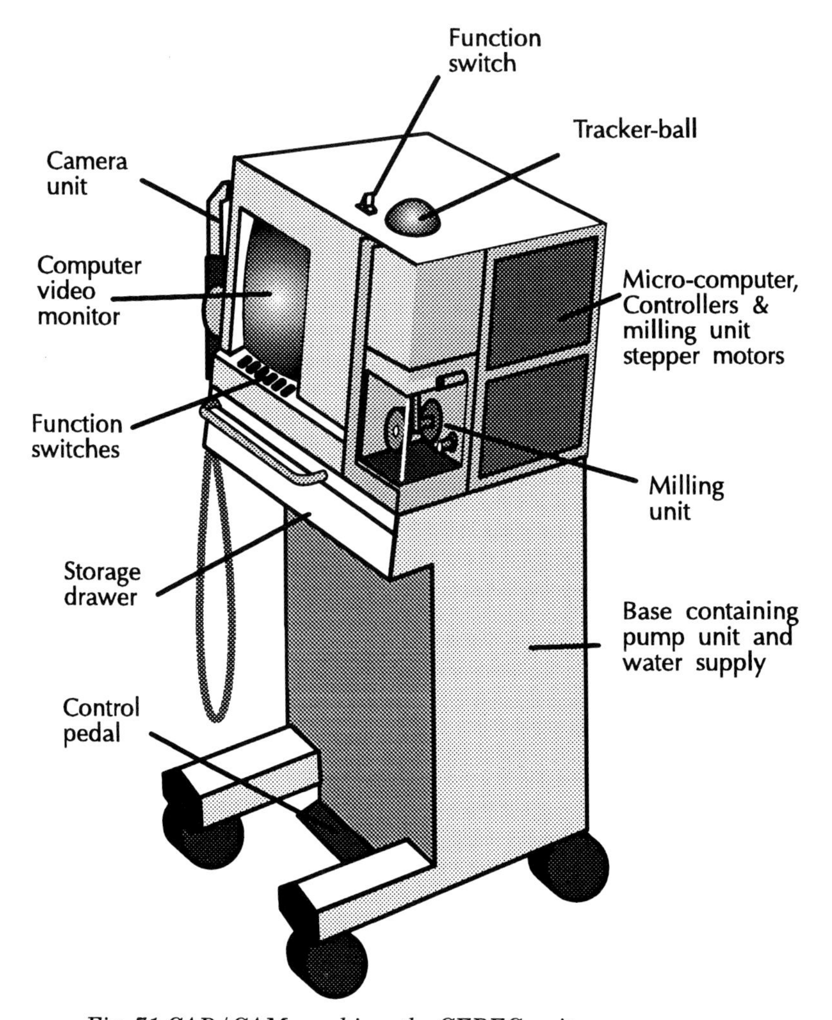

Fig. 71.CAD / CAM machine: the CEREC unit.

The 'CEREC' concept is the ingenious result of a sophisticated analysis of the requirements of a dental restorative system and the application of logical problem reduction. This is combined with an elegant and effective engineering solution, matched to the problem-reduction model.

The tooth preparation is rationalised to exclude the need for internal machining of the ceramic blank. This allows speedy production of the final restoration by a turbine-driven diamond milling disk in a single pass along the ceramic blank. The topography of the tooth preparation is recorded optically in a fraction of a second and a digital model created in the computer.

The optical impression

In order to make the surface of the tooth visible to the infra-red illuminator in the active camera, it is necessary to coat the tooth with titanium oxide powder. This highly-reflective powder is sprayed on as a dry dust. The tooth is first coated with a polysorbate film, the imaging liquid. This holds the powder in place.

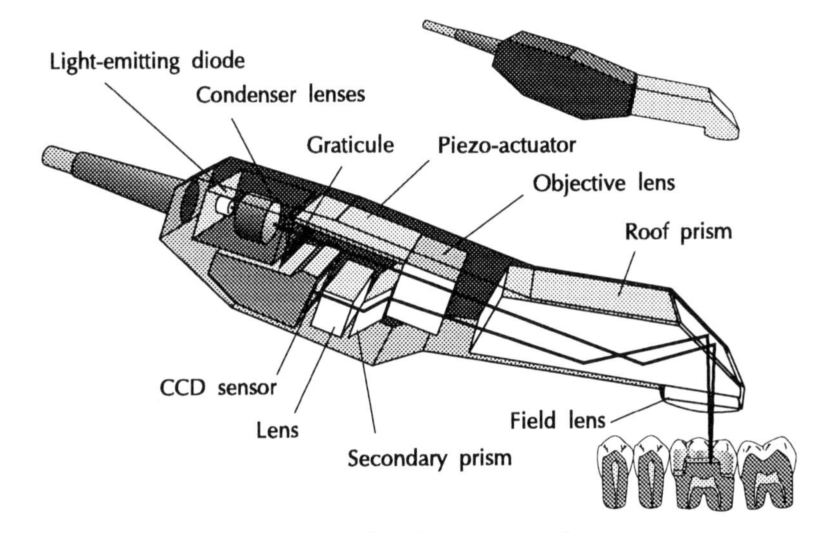

Fig. 72. Three-dimensional active camera unit.

The structure of the camera unit is shown in *Fig. 72*. A light emitting diode projects the image of a grid onto the tooth surface. The camera observes this grid from a slight angle. Vertical contour of the cavity is observed as a lateral shift in the lines of the grid brought about by a parallax effect. This shift is used to determine the physical measurement of height.

Software and the restoration design

Once a three-dimensional model of the tooth preparation is recorded the restoration must be designed on top of it. The first generation software required some level of design intervention by the operator but as the software has become more sophisticated less skill is needed. The operator maps out the base of the restoration by placing plotting points on the photograph of the cavity which appears on a computer monitor *(Fig. 73)*. The machine extrapolates across this area and determines the true topography of the cavity floor.

The operator next outlines the approximal surface and the machine suggests the placement of the marginal ridge. These features may be edited easily. The points are joined up by the computer which then locates the occlusal margin of the cavity using a wall-finding algorithm which looks progressively up the wall of the cavity until a horizon is located. It identifies this as the cavity edge *(Fig. 74)*. These data are used to construct a wire-frame model of the restoration. Editing of the data is possible to alter the external profile of the final restoration. The wire-frame model is stored to disk and the data are used to drive a milling machine which shapes a block of ceramic to the required form. After the volume model has been created, a ceramic block is inserted into the milling machine and the device renders the final restoration.

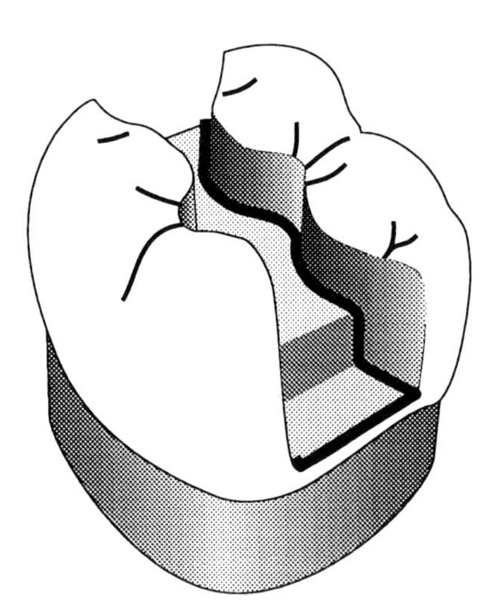

Fig. 73. The base of the cavity is outlined on the computer screen.

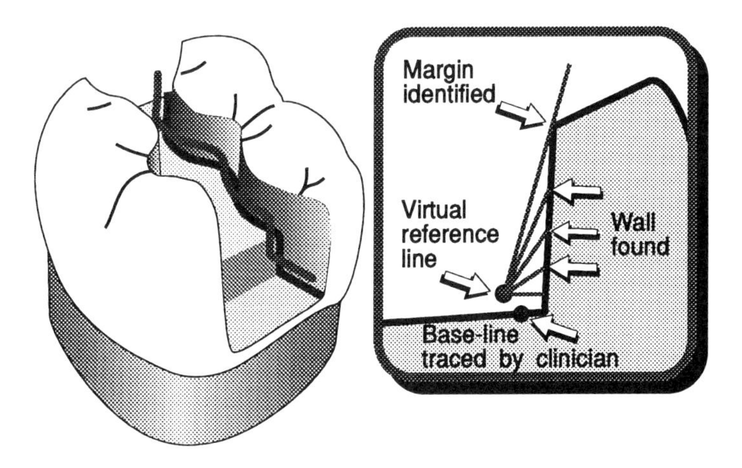

Fig. 74. The operation of the margin-locating algorithm.

The milling unit

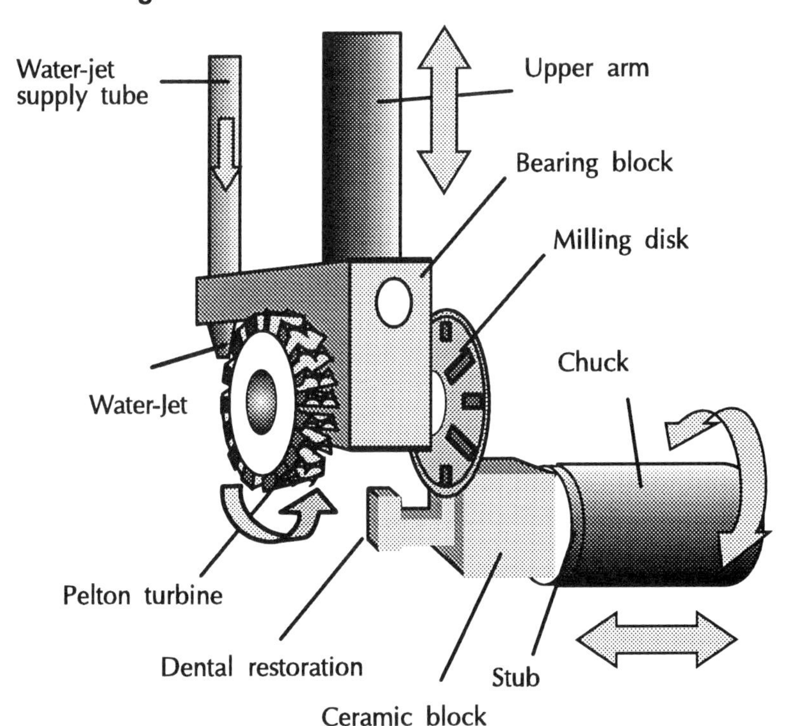

Fig. 75. Milling unit of the Siemens CEREC.

The milling machine is illustrated in *Fig. 75*. This is the original hydraulic turbine version. An electric drive is now available and provides a finer surface finish on the ceramic restoration and a much improved cutting efficiency.

Milling with a rotary disk is simple and effective but there are certain limitations of cut which are implicit in the system. The preparations cut in the tooth must be designed to take these limitations into account *(Fig. 76)*.

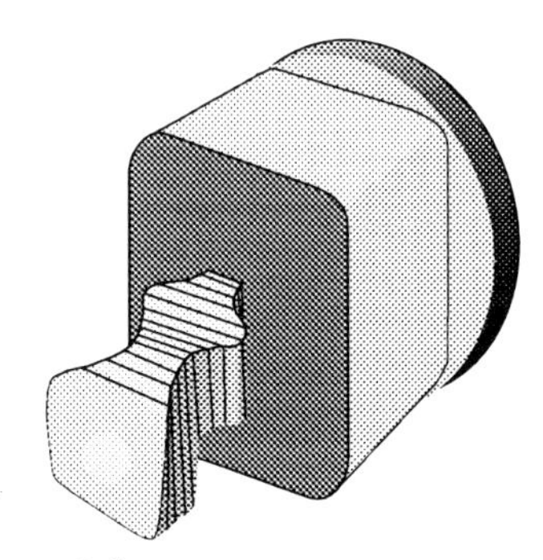

Fig. 76. A part-cut inlay.

Fig. 77 illustrates the range of shapes which may be made using a cutting disk in a rotary milling unit and some of the limitations.

Possible:

A: external curves in the plane of the cutting disk on any surface.

B: external curves perpendicular to the plane of the cutting disk on any surface.

C: straight steps across the whole of a surface in the plane of the cutting disk.

Not possible:

X: steps with risers at angles to the plane of the cutting disk.

Y: internal curves with a radius smaller than that of the cutting disk.

Z: undercut surfaces.

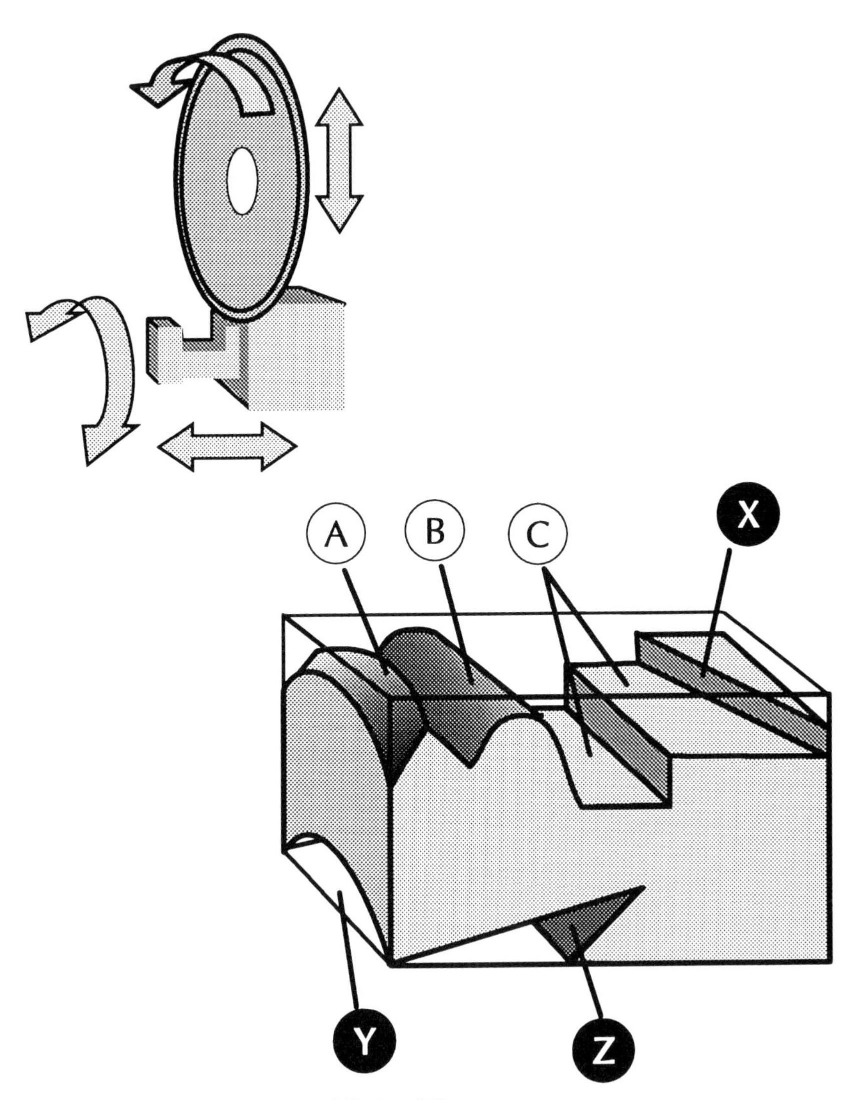

Fig. 77. Limitations of disk milling.

Steps in the same plane as the disk are not possible nor are any areas of internal milling such as would be needed to fabricate a crown. This limitation affects the design of cavity which can prepared. However, most cavity surfaces can be restored with modifications to the traditional cavity design.

Machining such a small item as a dental crown, bridge or inlay requires high levels of precision, especially when creating an internal fitting surface such as that of of crown. A capstan-head milling machine is needed to fabricate the inner surfaces of crowns as a number of cutting instruments will be needed to create the shape. Such machines take much greater time in manufacturing the restoration and this means that in the foreseeable future they are likely to be limited to laboratory use and will not allow single-visit crown placement. Cost appears to be the greatest obstacle to commercial realisation of working systems.

Laboratory-based CAD/CAM systems are available and mostly rely on digitising data from dental models which are cast from conventional impressions. The digitising systems are based on mechanical stylus tracing and this takes a considerable time to do.

It is more than reasonable to look at the direction in which technology is moving and predict that the next stage of tooth reconstruction which will come to the attention of the computer technologist is the cutting of the tooth preparations. In this way the machine could optimise all stages of rebuilding or replacing a tooth.

Structural analysis can be integrated into computer-aided design. This is known as finite element analysis or FEA. FEA allows the distribution of stresses in a structural design to be analysed. From this information the design of the structure can be modified in order to optimise the stress distribution both in the structure itself and in the structures which support it. Integrating such a design system into a dental CAD/CAM system is a formidable but achievable task which would allow the development of restorations far superior to any of today.

CHAPTER 9

Computer Systems

Computers and micro-processors are finding increasing use in dental practice. Apart from being used in their own right as computers for practice administration, many microcomputer devices are built into dental units and instrumentation for control purposes. Many combined dental chairs and instrument delivery systems use a dedicated micro-processor to control the operating functions. Devices such as radiovisiography can only be built because of the micro-processor.

Mainframe computers

A mainframe computer is a large central computer of the type used by banks or large companies. The major characteristic of a mainframe is that it can serve many hundreds of users simultaneously, and accommodate different tasks for each user. This is known as 'multi-user, multi-tasking'. However such functionality is no longer the preserve of mainframe computers and the more sophisticated desk-top computers can provide these services. Likewise, the massive data-storage facility of a mainframe can be achieved using optical disk systems in much smaller machines.

Dental practices are highly unlikely to have a mainframe computer installed on the premises but many will communicate with mainframe computers installed in the account-holder's bank, dental insurance and fee-paying agencies and other institutions.

Mini-computers

The term mini-computer is used to refer to computers which are intermediate in size between microcomputers and mainframes. As the power of smaller computers increases this becomes a very fuzzy definition because a sophisticated, top of the range personal computer can now outperform many so-called mini-computers of recent years. The best way of defining a mini-computer is one which is designed from the outset to support multiple users and multiple programs at the same time.

The personal computer

The personal computer or 'microcomputer' *(Figs 78–81)* was designed originally to support a single independent user working on a single task at a time. As the machines have grown in sophistication multi-tasking has become possible on these machines as has the support of several users simultaneously.

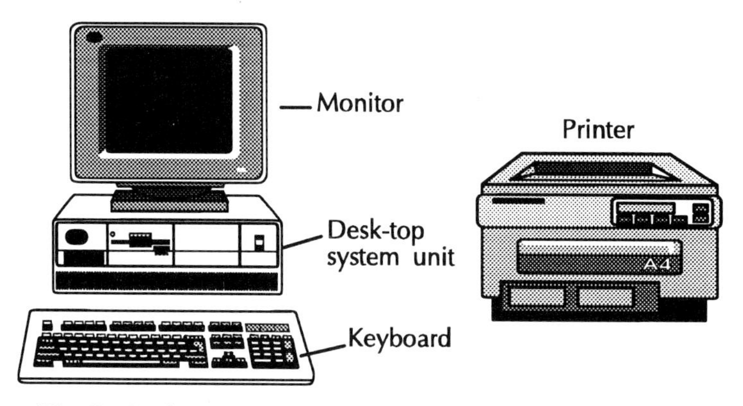

Fig. 78. Desk-top personal computer and printer.

The basic components of a microcomputer are the central processor chip, memory chips, disk storage for data, a keyboard and display monitor. The main difference between microcomputers is in the choice of central processor chip and in the architecture of the circuitry which supports it.

Business computing is dominated by the standards set by IBM in the 1980s with the introduction of their range of personal computers. The vast majority of personal computers used today follow this architecture. Several features have led to the large-scale adoption of this system. The IBM PC consists of a basic circuit board, known as the motherboard, which contains the microcomputer chip and associated circuitry. A number of slot-connectors on the motherboard enable a range of additional circuit boards to be added to the system. These boards include interfaces to disk drives, various standards of video monitor, special boards to drive printers or communicate with other computers and many others. This architecture enables each computer system to be customised for its particular purpose but still maintain overall compatibility with other computers of its type.

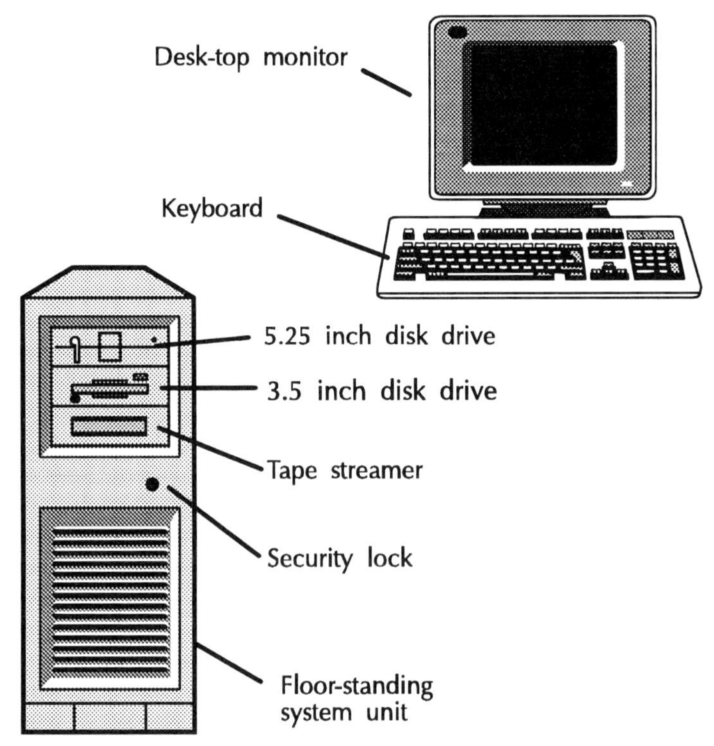

Fig. 79. Floor-standing personal computer.

The earliest IBM PCs were based on a microchip produced by Intel and known as the 8088. Since then the range has expanded through the 8086, 80186, 80286, 80386 and the 80486. Each chip being significantly more sophisticated than its predecessor yet still maintaining enough backwards compatibility to be able to run existing software. Machines based on all these processors are still manufactured and lead to a wide price range. For the software of today and the immediate future only machines based on 80386 chips or above should be considered for use in a dental practice.

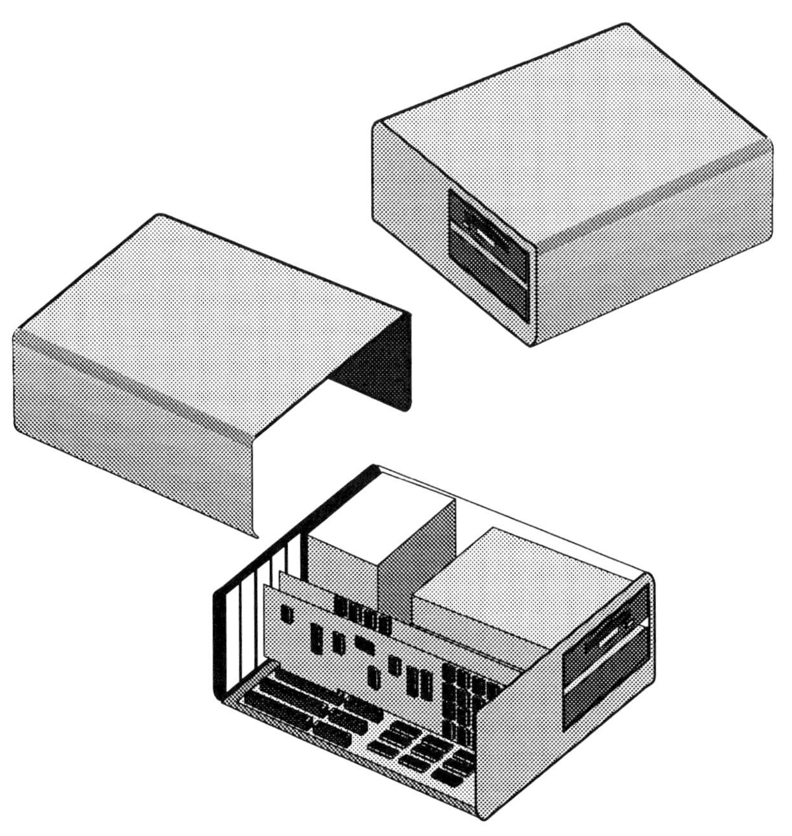

Fig. 80. Interior view of typical system unit.

One of the important features of microcomputers is the bus system. The bus is the internal interconnection system of the computer. The plug-in connector slots which enable the addition of various extra feature boards are connected to the bus and the bus determines the manner in which interconnection between these and the main system components occurs. Two main architectures now exist. The original bus architecture of the IBM PC has been developed into ISA (Industry Standard Architecture). IBM have moved to a standard known as micro-channel architecture. This latter standard finds wide acceptance because of its level of functionality and because of its pedigree with IBM. Micro-channel architecture allows multiple processors to co-exist on the same bus system. This allows very sophisticated desk-top computers indeed. Rival manufacturers have developed the ISA bus in a competitive manner to achieve many of the features of micro-channel architecture. This system is known as EISA (Extended Micro-Channel Architecture).

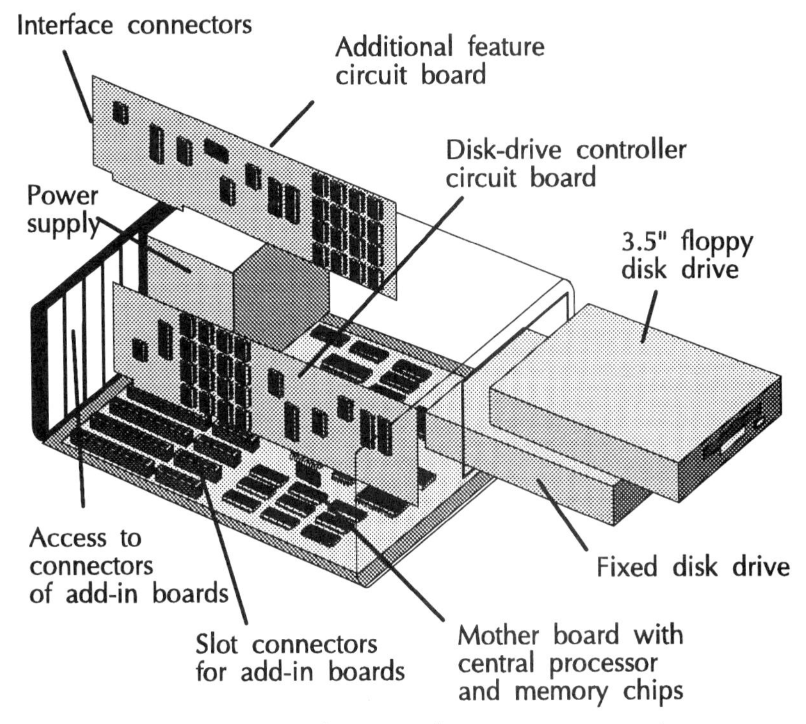

Fig. 81. Construction of a personal computer system unit.

Software

Operating systems

The operating system of a computer can be likened to a housekeeper. The operating system is a program which is responsible for the background management of the computer system and all its features whilst an applications program is running.

The major operating system for IBM-type personal computers is MS-DOS. (MicroSoft Disk Operating System), often referred to simply as DOS. This has its origins in 1980 but has seen massive upgrades since. Variants are produced by certain machine manufacturers to accommodate the idiosyncrasies of their particular machines. MS-DOS remains the most popular operating system and is likely to do so for many years to come. Like other programs, the upgrading versions of MS-DOS are identified by two numbers separated by a decimal point. The first number indicates the major revision number and the second indicates minor revisions of the version. MS-DOS 5.0 is the current version at the time of writing.

An alternative to DOS is Operating System 2 (OS/2). This was designed from the outset as a multi-tasking operating system and is suitable for larger personal computers.

Most operating systems require a significant knowledge of the system before they can be operated with ease. An alternative approach is to present information and programs graphically and this is implemented in Graphical User Interfaces (GUIs). The most popular GUI is marketed by Microsoft as Microsoft Windows. It is not a program in the sense that it has a specific function, but rather an overlay for the operating system whereby other programs may be run in a consistent graphical manner. Its main characteristic is its tremendous ease of use. People totally untrained in the use of a computer can start to use basic programs within hours rather than days. Furthermore, for the advanced user there are many other features of importance such as dynamic linking whereby one program is able to call on another for data, or is able to update data in another program without that program having been called by the operator. This means that if a patient address list is altered within a word-processing document, all references to that address which appear in other documents, even from other programs, are updated automatically. There is little doubt that the Windows interface will become the standard for the future.

An operating system which has spread down from mainframes and minicomputers is UNIX. There are several variations of this system which is usually a full multi-tasking, multi-user operating system. Whilst UNIX can be run on Intel 80x86 based machines, it is usually reserved for workstation computers, mini-computers and mainframes. Software for UNIX and its derivatives is generally much more costly than that for MS-DOS and there is a much narrower range of material available.

Applications software

Applications software is the term applied to the programs which are run on a computer. Each has a specific purpose or application.

Word-processors

A word-processor is a program which enables text to be typed, formatted and printed using a computer. Whilst a word-processor can be used for simple tasks such as typing a letter, its full value is found in more extensive documents such as this book. The entire book was written as a single document using the word-processor 'Microsoft Word'. Formatting, page layout, insertion and numbering of graphics, cross-referencing and indexing are all looked after by the word-processor.

Most word-processors incorporate a spell-checker and many have an on-line thesaurus. The most sophisticated have a grammar-checking function as well.

Spreadsheets

A spreadsheet is a sophisticated mathematical work-sheet viewed through the computer screen. The sheet is divided into cells similar to the squares on school mathematics paper. Data are entered into the cells in an analogous manner. Formulae are written to relate one or more cells together mathematically and the answer is displayed in another cell.

In this manner spreadsheets can be used to set up and calculate accounts, statistics or any other mathematical problem.

Databases

Databases are used for storing series of data. For example, names and addresses of patients, details of recalls, records of treatment given, etc. The data can then be accessed and processed in a manner prescribed by the computer operator. For example, all patients requiring recall in any particular month can be listed.

Integrated packages

Many programs are now available which serve all the functions of a word-processor, a spreadsheet and a database. Such programs are often referred to as integrated packages.

Presentation graphics

Computers are very useful for creating graphics for presentation purposes. Data and results from spreadsheet calculations can be depicted graphically and the resulting image printed onto a transparency for an overhead projector or a 35 mm slide. Illustration programs can create pictures and these can be printed to transparency, slide or paper. Presentation graphics packages assist even the most artistically incompetent to produce acceptable presentation slides by providing templates upon which text and data can be superimposed.

Design and illustration

Programs which provide drawing tools and sizing grids allow the production of drawings and designs ranging from the simple to the complex. The great advantage of such programs is that once an illustration is created it can be edited, re-sized and re-coloured to suit many purposes. For example, the same graphic can be used to produce a colour slide or to illustrate a textbook. All the illustrations in this book were created directly on a computer using a sophisticated illustration program.

Desk-top publishing

Desk-top publishing programs are an advance on word-processing, allowing advanced manipulation of page layouts, typographical design and graphic image editing. The borderline between word-processing and desk-top publishing is becoming increasingly ill-defined.

Practice management programs

Specific programs are now available to assist in the business of operating a dental practice. Many programs are obtainable and offer a wide range of functions and options, ranging from simple database work to fully integrated patient record and accounting systems.

Communication packages

Communication programs are designed to allow one computer to interchange information with another. This may be over a telephone line using a modem (page 121) or over other communication lines. Communication programs may be used for making enquiries of remote databases, for downloading data from a remote computer or for simply linking two computers within one practice.

Storing information

Removable magnetic disks

Computer systems need to store programs and data. The earliest computers used punched cards or punched paper tape. Today the vast majority of data storage is accomplished with magnetic disks of various types. Removable disks are usually flexible and store limited amounts of data. Several standards of floppy disk exist *(Fig. 82)*. The original standard was a flexible magnetic disk contained in a soft 5.25 inch jacket. The formats of the disk included 160 kilobytes, 320 kb, 360 kb and 1.2 Megabytes. The 5.25 inch disk is being replaced with disks held in rigid 3.5 inch plastic containers and formatted to 720 kb or 1.44 Mb. The disk density can be identified by the presence of a small aperture at the top left of the plastic disk case. The aperture at the right side is a write-protect switch to prevent accidental overwriting of valuable data. When a small slider which blocks the aperture is opened, the disk can only be read. 2.88 Mb format and higher have also been introduced. These disks are more convenient and considerably less vulnerable than the 5.25 inch disks.

Magnetic disks require careful handling and storage. They should be kept dry and should not be exposed to extremes of temperature. Above all, they must be protected from magnetic fields. Stray magnetic fields from electric motors, loudspeakers and other devices are all capable of damaging the data stored on disks. Pocket dictation machines often have powerful magnets in the speakers and motors and can erase data from a floppy disk.

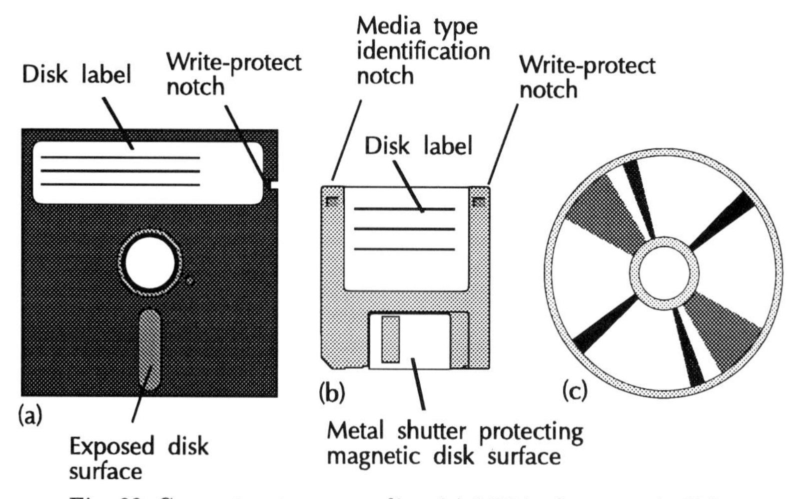

Fig. 82. Computer storage media. (a) 5.25 inch magnetic disk; (b) 3.5 inch magnetic disk; (c) 12 cm optical disk (CD ROM).

Hard magnetic disk drives

To achieve a higher level of storage the disks must be finely surfaced and extremely stable. This can only be done by using a number of rigid disks sealed in a dust-proof enclosure. These are known as 'hard disk drives' *(Fig. 83)* and on average store 50 to 500 times the amount of information contained on a removable floppy disk. The metal, or sometimes ceramic, recording disks in the drive rotate at 3000 rpm. Read-write heads are suspended close to, but not in contact with, the disk surface and are swept laterally across the disk to access information. The movement of the arm across the disk is actuated by a stepper motor. This is a special kind of motor which rotates in fixed steps, often 256 to a circle. Each step requires one electromagnetic pulse within the windings of the motor. By sending the correct number of forward or reverse pulses to the motor, the arms can be positioned rapidly and accurately over the disk surface. The geometry of the swept pattern on the surface of the disk is known as the disk format. The concentric rings of data are known as tracks and sections of each track are known as sectors. Each concentric ring or track will have a matched opponent on the other side of the disk and on the two sides of the adjacent disk. These vertically aligned tracks are known as cylinders.

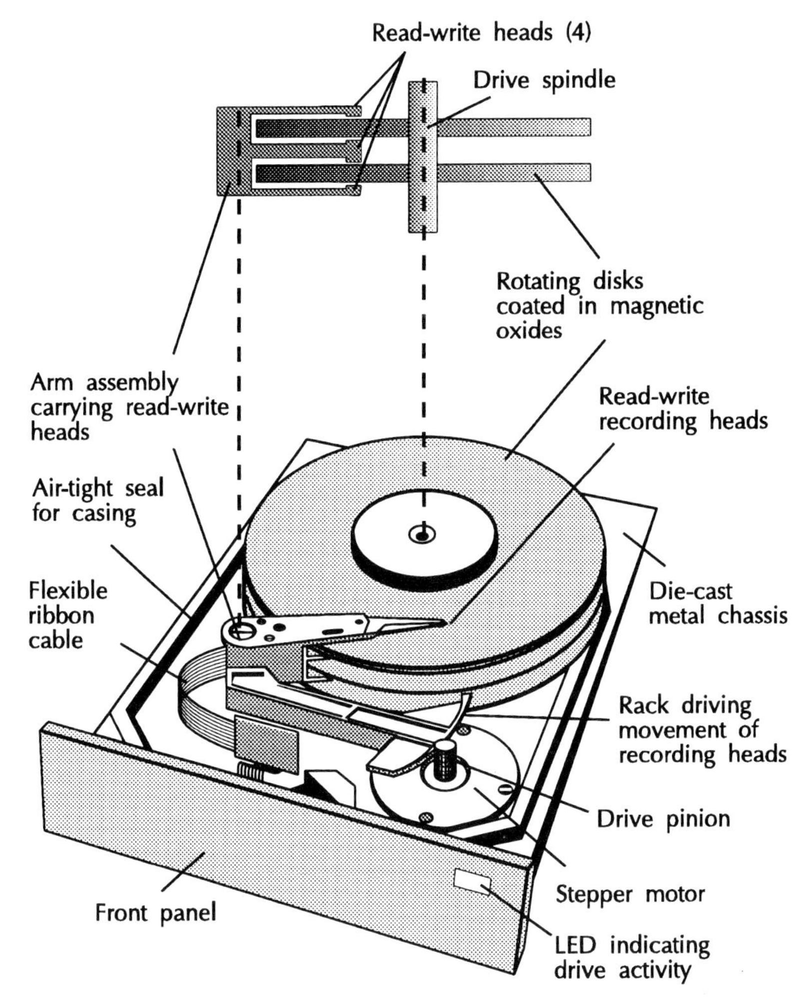

Fig. 83. Typical hard disk drive with cover removed to show the read-write heads and recording disks. This particular unit records on four disk surfaces. The heads move across the disk in the manner of a pick-up arm over a gramophone record.

One significant danger of using large hard disks is that large amounts of data can be lost if back-up copies are not created and maintained with the highest discipline. Back-up devices add significantly to the cost of computer systems and are often neglected in what becomes futile cost-saving.

Optical disk drives

Optical disk drives provide storage for vast quantities of information running into the range of hundreds of gigabytes. Such systems have application in dental practices for large total record systems. Optical disks generally have slower access times than magnetic drives but are becoming faster as the technology improves.

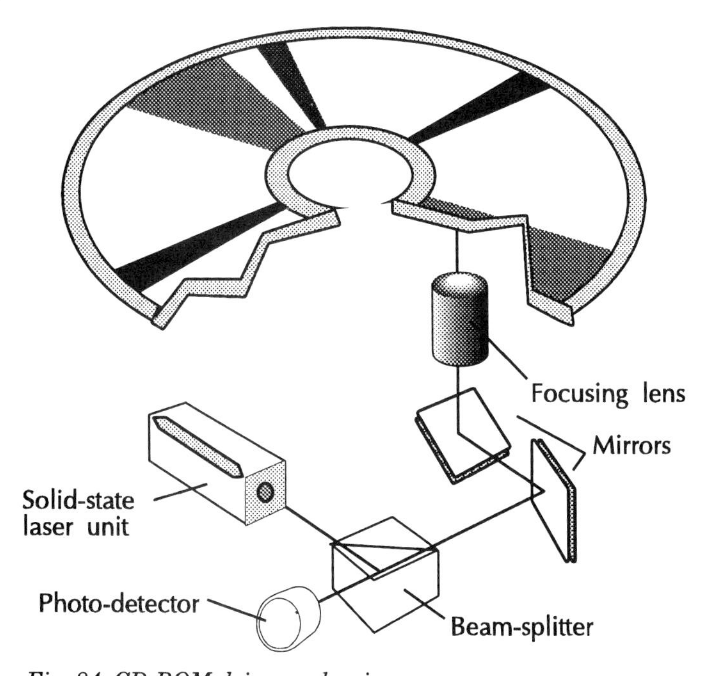

Fig. 84. CD-ROM drive mechanism.

Three major types of optical drives are manufactured. The first is a read-only version known as CD-ROM. CD-ROM drives read information encoded on compact discs, similar to those used for sound recording. These allow a publisher to produce a vast amount of information on a single source and are used mainly for works of reference. The data are recorded in the form of minute pits and grooves in a reflective surface within a transparent plastic disk. A laser beam illuminates the pits and is modulated upon reflection *(Fig. 84)*. The modulated beam carrying the information passes through a beam-splitting prism and is detected by a photo-sensitive transistor.

WORM drives, (Write Once, Read Many) allow writing of data only once; ie. the data, once written, cannot be erased or altered. Such drives have large volume capacity which makes them useful for archival purposes.

The third variety of optical disk drive allows writing, reading and erasing of data. These function in a manner analogous to magnetic disks and are the most versatile form of optical data storage. In principle, data recorded on such disks is more secure than that written to magnetic disks. Re-writeable optical disks can store large volumes of data and can operate at speeds approaching a slow hard magnetic disk drive.

Back-up systems

It is vital that a copy is kept of all important data so that if the system fails the data can be restored. Making back-up copies of data on hard disks can be a tedious and time-consuming process. The easiest way is to have the process automated by running time-triggered back-up programs which operate out of hours. Back-up copies can be made onto tape cassettes using devices known as tape-streamers.

Another way to operate a back-up system is to have two identical hard disk systems operating in tandem so that one drive shadows the other. If the primary drive fails then the shadow drive takes over without any interruption of data storage or the need to restore information from back-up disks. Personal computers are available with this feature built in.

Printers

Printers can be divided into two groups, impact printers and non-impact printers. Impact printers use a mechanical action to strike an inked ribbon against the paper. Non-impact printers create the image on the paper in other ways such as squirting ink directly or heating a sensitive coating on the paper.

In most cases, impact printers are cheapest to buy and cheapest to run. The ribbons last for a considerable period and fail slowly with plenty of time to order a replacement.

The main advantage of non-impact printers is the relatively low noise of operation. This has obvious importance in a dental practice where such background noise can be most disturbing.

Impact printers

Dot-matrix printers

Dot-matrix printers operate by striking a ribbon against the printing paper with a number of fine metal pins *(Fig. 85)*. These points are arranged vertically to a height spanning one line of print. Basic models use nine pins, better quality printers use 24 pins and achieve a higher resolution.

Dot-matrix impact printers are fast, cheap and noisy. They are useful for long print-runs in an office environment where background noise is acceptable. For example, they are useful for producing cheap circulars which may be printed overnight whilst the office is empty. For most other purposes there are better printers available.

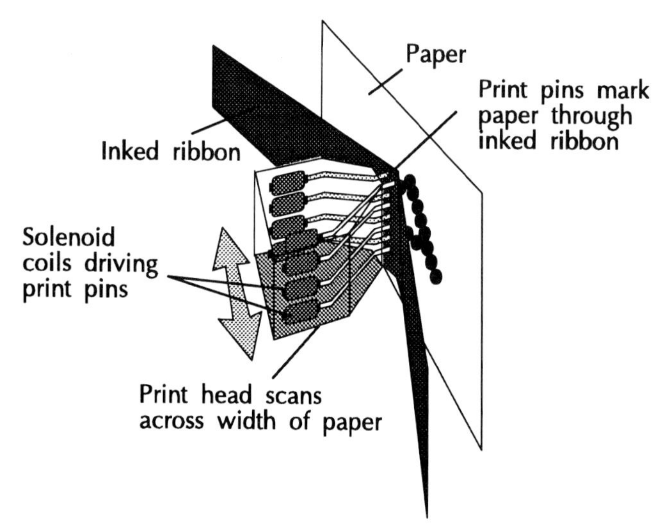

Fig. 85. Print head of a dot-matrix impact printer.

Daisy-wheel printers

Daisy-wheel printers are really just a modification of the daisy-wheel typewriter. Printing letters are arranged on the spokes of a wheel which may be rotated to bring any character in alignment between a hammer and the paper. The hammer strikes the spoke bearing the selected letter and this creates an inked image on the paper through an intervening ribbon.

The print quality of a daisy-wheel printer is excellent, but is limited to text. Graphics cannot be handled easily although some printers try to achieve crude images by building up the image from period marks. Daisy-wheels are noisy in operation but cheap to run. They have a role where high quality print appearance is needed at minimal cost but there is a tremendous penalty in the volume of noise generated.

Non-impact printers

Ink-jet printers

Ink-jet printers have been developed to a high level and the best machines can match the print output quality of an average laser printer. Ink-jet printers operate by spitting small dots of ink directly onto the paper. A density of 300 dots per inch can be achieved with modern machines. The only noise is from the transport of the printing head across the paper and from the transport of paper through the machine. The actual printing head is virtually silent. These machines are highly reliable, give an excellent quality of output and are generally much cheaper to run than a laser printer. Large amounts of memory in the printer are not needed because the device can accept data line-by-line from the computer. Provided the computer can calculate a full-page graphic image, the printer can print it. This makes high quality graphic printing relatively cheap.

However, they are not capable of high-speed printing and are not suited to massive print-runs. Apart from printing out circulars and other long runs, ink-jet printers serve the needs of a dental practice very well.

Colour ink-jets are about the cheapest and most cost-effective route into colour printing. Resolutions up to 300 dots per inch of printed area are available and the colour images produced can be quite stunning. However, the speed of printing is correspondingly much lower than monochrome systems and can be as low as one page every 20 minutes for complex graphics.

Thermal printers

Thermal printers operate with either special thermal ribbon or print directly to a thermally-sensitive coated paper. Some machines may work in either mode.

A network of pins form the letters by heating briefly and causing a darkening of the sensitive paper. Where a ribbon is used it is pressed firmly against the paper and the ink from the ribbon is melted onto the paper surface.

Thermal printers use little electricity and are therefore very suitable for use in portable machines. However, running costs are usually high due to the need to buy expensive coated paper or special ribbons which can be used once only. Thermal printers printing to coated paper are the usual printing output system in fax machines.

Laser printers

Laser printers offer the best quality and highest speed output of any printers today *(Fig. 86)*. However there is a penalty for this in terms of complexity of construction and cost of operation.

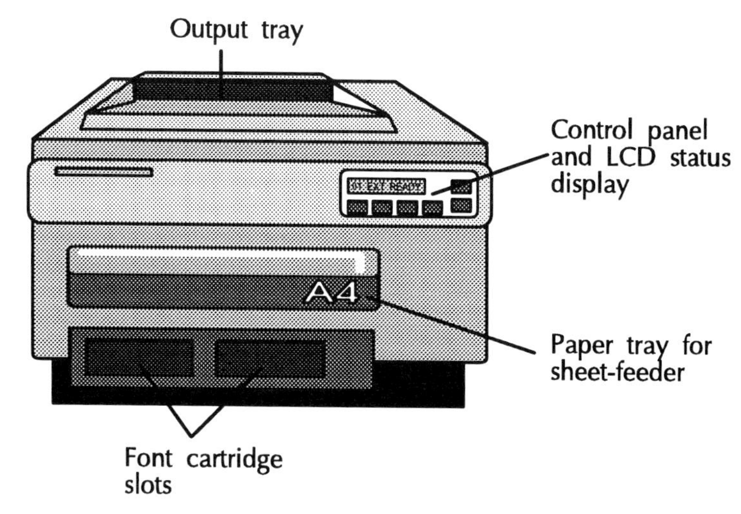

Fig. 86. A typical laser printer.

Laser printers operate by creating an image of the page to be printed on an electrostatic drum. This is done by charging the surface of the drum with a high voltage and then scanning the surface with a laser. The scan discharges areas of the drum selectively. A fine toner powder is then attracted to the drum where the electrostatic charge remains. This powder is then transferred to the surface of the printing paper by reversing the charge so that the powder sticks to the paper. The paper then passes between heated rollers and the toner powder is melted onto its surface. A very high resolution image results.

The need to scan the whole image of the page onto the drum at the same time means that enough memory must be fitted into the printer to achieve this. At a resolution of 300 dots per inch (dpi) one megabyte of memory is needed to print an A4 page of graphics. This heavy demand for RAM chips increases the cost of the printers significantly.

Desk-top laser printers and printer enhancement accessories allow resolutions of 600 dpi and some machines can reach 1200 dpi which is entering the realms of photo type-setting machines.

Printer control languages

In order to drive more sophisticated printers a range of printer control languages have been developed. The most sophisticated of these is Postscript which was developed by Adobe Systems Inc. This language is known as a 'page description language' because it communicates a full description of the page to be printed to the printer before printing is commenced. A wide range of word-processors and graphics packages now support this standard. One draw-back of Postscript is that the printer requires a Postscript controller card and a considerable amount of memory. This, together with the licensing costs in manufacture, make Postscript printers very expensive.

Hewlett-Packard have developed their own printer control language which is known as Hewlett-Packard Graphic Language or HPGL. This has developed through several versions and is used over a wide range of printers ranging from laser printers to graphic plotters. It is supported by a wide range of software and has become a standard emulated in printers from other manufacturers. It does not require the hardware overhead of Postscript although in laser printers it can make use of several megabytes of memory if available.

Scanners

Optical scanners are devices which allow text or graphics to be scanned optically and a digital image to be created and stored in the computer. Scanners can be either hand-held or desk-top units. Pictures can be scanned in to be incorporated into desk-top publishing documents, or to be modified with graphics programs. Typed script can be scanned and the text read by optical character recognition (OCR) programs. In this way, a document which has been prepared on a conventional typewriter can be fed into a computer and edited with a word-processor program without the tedious and expensive process of copy typing.

Larger installations

Single-user microcomputers have limited use. When the dentist needs to expand his system and have access from several points around the practice then a multi-user system is necessary. It becomes important to access the same database from the surgery and from the reception area. There are two ways of achieving this, one single computer can be used to support a number of terminals or a number of computers can be linked together using a network.

Multi-user, multi-tasking computers

A multi-user single computer system is illustrated in *Fig. 87*. It is the cheapest solution but does have a number of disadvantages. Firstly, the whole system depends on the single computer and its subsystems. If this goes down then the whole system is inoperable. Secondly, the host computer must divide its attention across the number of terminals which are seeking it. A terminal has no intrinsic processing capability and is used only to communicate with the host computer. If the tasks become complex over a number of terminals then the response time of the computer may be unacceptably long. Certainly, high-resolution graphic interfaces cannot be supported in this manner.

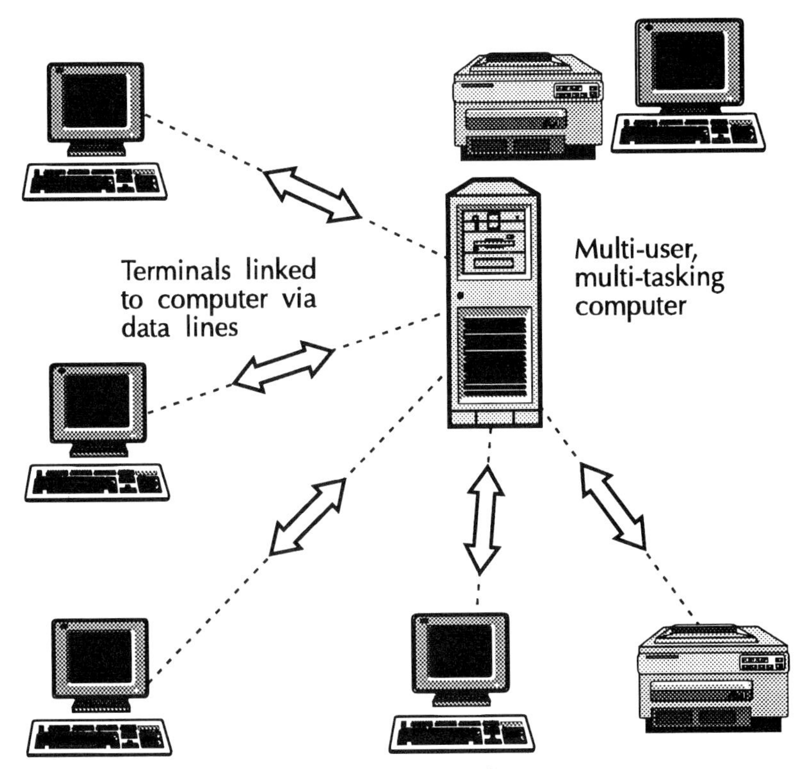

Fig. 87. Multi-user, multi-tasking single computer system.

Networked computer systems

The alternative to a single, shared computer is to use a network to link a number of personal computers together. In this way, the requirements of each work-place may be catered for in full but communal information may be accessed by any machine. Two major networking standards exist, EtherNet and Token Ring. One of the strongest systems is the token ring network. The layout of this technology is illustrated in *Fig. 88*. In this system each computer operates independently of the network but can call on the resources of the network at any time. Furthermore, if any single unit on the ring fails then it is switched out automatically and the network continues to operate undamaged. If key tasks such as shared printing are being performed by one of the units which fails then its activity can be reassigned to another node in the ring. This depends on the same facilities existing in the substitute node, but this can often be achieved by taking the printer down the corridor to a working node and plugging it in.

One unit of the node is usually assigned the job of acting as file-server. This unit is fitted with a high-speed, large capacity hard disk and provides programs and data to other nodes on the network. The network benefits from the installation of a high performance machine for this task.

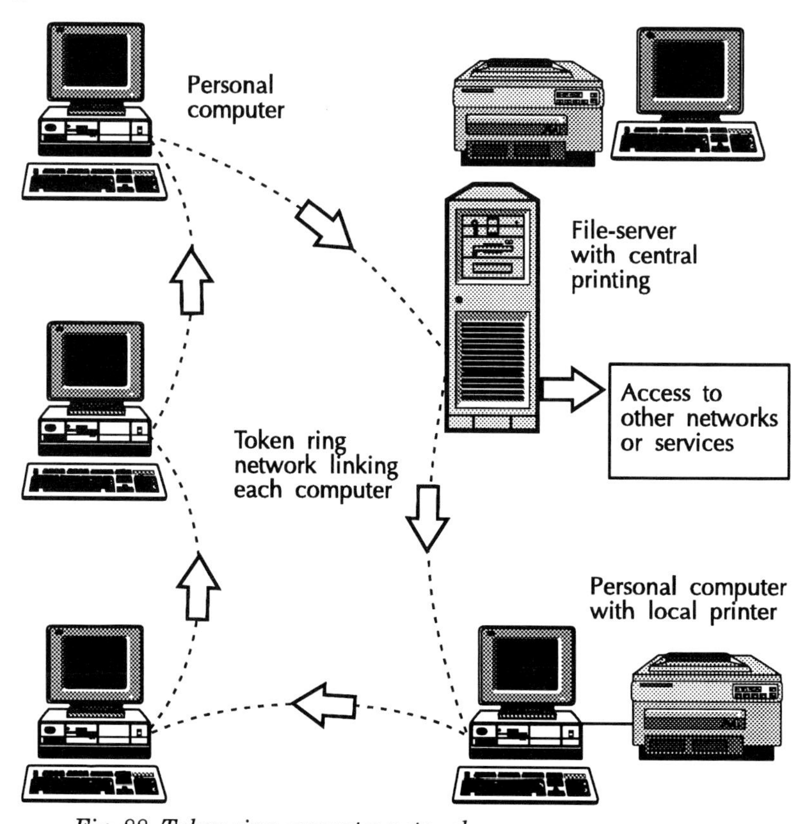

Fig. 88. Token ring computer network.

The token ring concept operates by passing an electronic code, or token from one computer to another around the circle. If any computer wants to send data around the ring then it modifies this token with its own address and the address of the recipient computer. Data is attached and the token sent around the ring. The recipient computer recognises its address on the token and accepts the data whilst other computers on the ring ignore it. Having accepted the data, the recipient computer switches the token back to its unoccupied state and puts it back on the ring for the next user to pick up when required.

Very large rings can be constructed using this system and many rings can be interconnected to create enormous networks. This makes the token-ring system very versatile and effective.

Modems

Communication between distant computers can be achieved over normal telephone lines. The data has to be encoded into a series of audio tones which can be transmitted over the telephone system in the same way as the voice. The device which produces the tones and which also receives incoming data in such a manner is known as a modem. A number of formats for these data links have been established by various international telecommunication administrative bodies. The standard formats, or communication protocols, which any particular modem is designed for are stated in the modem specification. Modems may be connected directly to the telephone system by direct wiring through a telephone socket or they can be connected to any telephone receiver by means of two pads, one a loudspeaker and one a microphone, through which the data tones are sent and received. Modems are usually attached to the computer through its serial communications port but sometimes they are built as slot-in extension cards.

Modems are one of the main methods of communicating between mainframe computers and personal computers. Data services may be either restricted to a single organisation or may be sold to specialist users. Many note-book computers have built-in modems to allow communication back to the main office computer when on location.

Some modems may be used for the transmission of fax data. In this way, a personal computer can send a fax directly over the public telephone network without having to print it out on paper and feed it through a fax machine (see page 128).

Power supplies

Most computer installations are extremely susceptible to problems with the mains electricity power supply. The mains supply is often contaminated with interference which may affect the operation of a computer. This interference may be in the form of spikes or surges of power when the supply voltage rises momentarily to very high levels. This can alter the contents of the computer memory or cause physical damage to circuits if it is severe enough. Spikes and surges may be introduced into the supply by heavy machinery switching in or out of the circuit or by other installations such as fluorescent lights. Another form of interference is superimposed radio-frequency interference. This may originate from devices such as wireless intercom systems and may affect computers in a manner similar to spikes.

Many forms of interference can be supressed or filtered out from the mains supply by using protected mains outlet sockets or plugs. Basic filters consist of inductors which filter out radio interference, combined with varistors to supress spikes. Varistors are wired across the supply cables and are normally non-conducting. When a certain voltage level is exceeded they become conducting and short out the voltage spike as it is rising. Instantly the voltage drops to its original level they become non-conducting again and the power resumes.

Uninterruptible power supplies

Unexpected loss of power can be disastrous within a computer system. Power loss may be due to a failure of the mains supply to the building or to fuses blowing within the circuit supplying a computer. An example of this problem is an air-compressor which faults out and fuses the circuit supplying other machines including the surgery computer.

Interruptions of power supplies to computers can be very damaging. At best, data which is live in the computer at the time is lost. At worst, the information stored on the disk drives can be corrupted. The latter occurs if the machine is trying to write to the disk when the power supply fails. It may be necessary to re-format the hard disk and re-install all the software and data from back-up copies.

The problems of power failure may be avoided by installing an uninterruptible power supply into the system. Uninterruptible power supplies consist of a back-up battery pack and automatic charging circuits together with a device which monitors the mains supply. The latter device switches in the batteries instantly when the supply fails, ensuring an uninterrupted supply of electricity to the computer.

Two types of uninterruptible power supply may be installed. Small units are designed to allow correct shut-down of the computer system so that damage does not occur. Larger units may allow the system to be used continuously for a considerable period until the supply is restored. The battery packs in such systems vary considerably in size and some may only be able to maintain the electrical supply for around 20 minutes or less. It is important that if a small unit is fitted there is an alarm system so that as soon as the uninterruptible power supply switches in the computer system can be shut down correctly, all files being closed and programs ended.

Film recorders

High quality slides for presentation purposes are best made on a purpose-built computer film recorder although photographing the screen is possible (see Chapter 11). These devices print a colour image directly on a normal colour transparency film. They are specified according the resolution of the image they can print and the number of colours in the image. Resolution is measured in terms of the number of discernable lines which can be printed on the film. Resolutions up to 8000 lines are available although units capable of this definition are very costly. The minimum resolution which would warrant the purchase of a film recorder rather than photographing directly from the screen is about 2000 lines. Many film recorders can achieve 16.7 million colours and this also adds significantly to the quality and impact of the recorded image. Special software is needed to take advantage of these recorders and purchasers need to ensure that their particular graphics software is able to take advantage of the high specification features of the film recorder.

Film recorders usually produce the image on a high resolution cathode-ray tube and then focus the image optically onto the film through either a dedicated camera back or in-built lens system. The cathode ray tube is monochrome because this allows for the highest levels of definition. Colour is formed by making three separate and sequential exposures through red, green and blue filters. Each exposure can take a considerable period of time.

CHAPTER 10

Communications

Communications play a major role in the effective running of any dental practice. Increasingly practices are providing out of hours emergency services and reliable contact between the dentist and his practice is necessary. Effective telephone systems, answering machines, radio paging systems and facsimile communications are becoming an essential part of practice life.

Telephone systems

The change from hard-wired systems to socketed telephones has created an enormous industry in added-feature telephones and accessories. Many of these have applications in dental practice.

Automatic dialling of frequently used numbers is a feature of many telephones but for a dental practice a separate autodialler may be very useful. This allows up to 100 pre-set numbers to be dialled at the touch of two buttons.

Loudspeaker telephones are helpful for the operatory where they allow two-way hands-free communication. This allows the dentist to receive calls without having to re-scrub to handle a telephone handset. Such telephones nearly always give the option of normal handset operation for confidential calls.

Public access branch exchanges may be used in larger practices where several telephone extensions are in use. This allows internal communication between telephones and the sharing of one or more external lines between all the extensions.

Radio pagers

Radio pagers provide a simple and relatively inexpensive method for a dentist to keep in touch with his practice. A radio pager is a small pocket-sized radio receiver which listens in constantly for a transmission of its identity code. When it receives this code it alerts the user by sounding a tone. Several forms are available ranging from simple tone pagers to full remote messaging systems.

Simple tone pagers emit a single tone bleep when a telephone number is dialled to alert the dentist. More sophisticated tone pagers have a range of tones to indicate which telephone called, for example, office or home.

Numeric pagers receive and display a number which is usually that of the telephone to be called in reply to the page. This type of pager may be accessed directly by telephoning its number followed by the number which is to appear on the pager screen.

Message pagers receive a short text message which is displayed on a two or more line screen on the pager. Most agencies who operate such a system have an operator who receives pager requests by voice and then transcribes the message to the paging transmitter.

Cellular telephones

Cellular telephone systems allow telephone calls to be transmitted and received through portable radio telephones. The cellular transmission system enables efficient use to be made of a limited range of transmission frequencies so that many telephones can use the system simultaneously. Each area of the country is divided into a large number of local cells. Within each cell the full range of available frequencies can be used. It is important that adjacent cells do not use the same frequency at the same time to avoid cross-channel interference. This means that in big cities the cells are relatively small to allow a high density of users whilst in the country the cells will be very much larger. Allocation of frequency is undertaken by a computer system which optimises the use of the network.

Portable telephones which work on the cellular networks range from built-in car telephones to tiny personal telephones which can be carried easily in a handbag or jacket pocket. The cost of the telephone itself is no longer very high, the greatest cost comes from the network rental and the cost of calls made over the network.

Answering machines

Telephone answering machines have become ubiquitous within business and extremely common in domestic houses. Simple machines use a single cassette tape to record both outgoing and incoming messages. This causes a delay after the outgoing message whilst the tape rewinds ready to record the incoming message. Better machines use either a separate tape or a solid state memory chip to record the outgoing message and this avoids any delays to the caller. Some machines incorporate voice synthesis circuits which record the date and time of the incoming call on the message tape. This is a very useful feature for dental practices.

Some more sophisticated machines will automatically dial out after a message is received so that a remote tone pager can be signalled to let the dentist know that there is a message waiting on the answerphone.

Facsimile communications

Direct transmission of page images from one site to another over a conventional telephone line is known as facsimile transmission or more colloquially as 'fax'. Sometimes the term 'telecopying' is used.

Fax machines have become ubiquitous within businesses. They allow near instant transmission of a document from one location to another and verification of a successful transmission, although the operation of the recipients' printer cannot be guaranteed. In terms of cost, it can be much cheaper to send a short document over a telephone line using a fax machine than to use the postal services. The appearance and layout of a typical fax machine is illustrated in *Fig. 89* and the mechanism is depicted in *Fig. 90.*

Fax machines scan the document to be transmitted and encode the data into a series of tone pulses which can be transmitted over a conventional telephone line. The document to be transmitted is placed into a tray on the top of the machine and is drawn slowly past an optical scanning head. The scanning mechanism sends the image line by line to the encoding circuitry where it is converted into a series of audio tones.

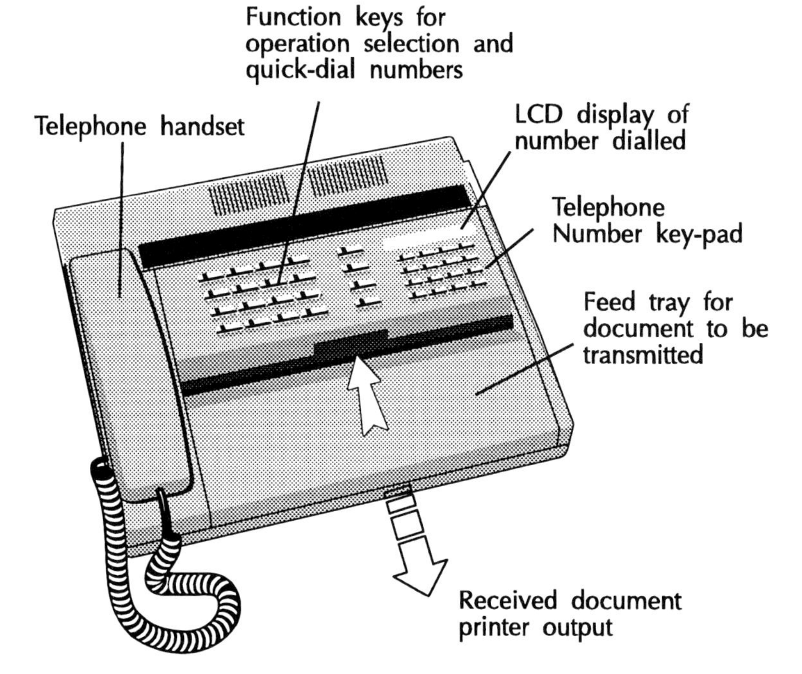

Fig. 89. External appearance and layout of a typical fax machine.

The audio tones are sent into the telephone network and are received by the other fax machine. The recipient machine decodes and prints each line of data as it is received using a thermal printer. In this manner, as the transmitted document passes under the scanner, the received copy is delivered virtually simultaneously *(Fig. 91)*. More sophisticated machines are capable of storing images in memory and printing them out later. This is especially useful if a confidential document is sent. It can only be printed out when an appropriate code is entered into the receiving machine by the addressee.

Fax machines follow well-defined communications standards. These standards cover image transmission at various levels of resolution and fax machines are available with several options in terms of transmission and reception. Simple machines allow for high/low definition switching. The most advanced machines have a grey-scale and half-toning function to allow the clear transmission of photographic images. Because only a limited bandwidth is available on telephone systems, transmission of extended-resolution images takes much longer with a consequent increase in telephone costs.

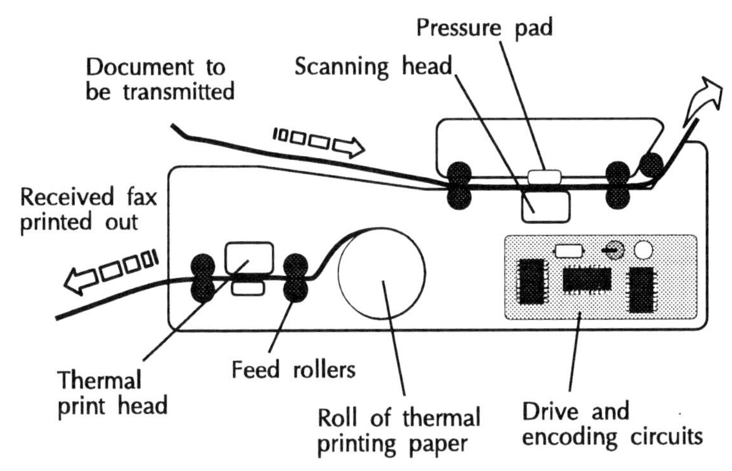

Fig. 90. Mechanism of a typical fax machine.

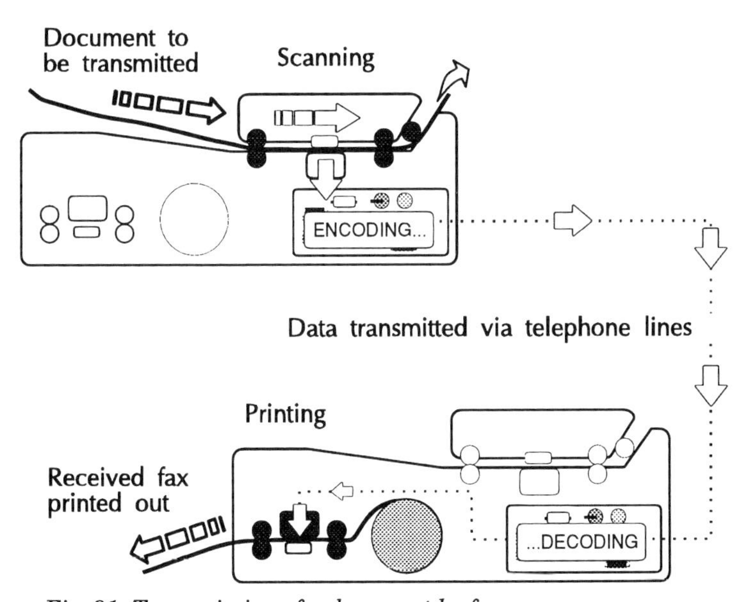

Fig. 91. Transmission of a document by fax.

Fax cards, or fax modems, are available for direct installation into a computer. This enables the fax function to be accessed directly from the computer keyboard. It is no longer necessary to print the document out on paper and then scan it; the encoding and data transmission can be done automatically as soon as a letter has been completed on the word-processor. Some fax boards allow reception as well as transmission of documents. This has the advantage that they can be printed out on normal paper on a laser printer rather than the somewhat transient thermal paper which is normally used in fax machines. A fax modem can be installed in a notebook computer allowing the business person to send faxes whilst away from the office.

One of the disadvantages of a fax machine used to be that it required a separate telephone line if calls were to be received unattended. Whilst this still remains the most convenient method of operation, it is no longer essential and a single line can be used for all purposes. A small control unit can be installed and connected to the normal telephone, the fax machine, a telephone answering machine and even a computer modem. When a call is received the device will automatically answer the telephone and listen for the characteristic tone of a transmitting fax unit. If this is received the telephone line will be connected to the fax unit. If not, the call will be sent to the normal telephone or the answerphone as appropriate with minimal delay to the caller.

Fax machines are now so commonplace that the critical mass of installations necessary to make the purchase of the machine a viable proposition is now long passed. Dental practices can certainly benefit from the installation of a fax machine, especially for ease and speed of communication with dental laboratories and suppliers of consumable items.

CHAPTER 11

Photographic Equipment

Photography is becoming an essential part of many dental practices today. Clinical photographs are used for pre-treatment and post-treatment patient records. These are useful for medico-legal purposes, patient education and motivation, staff education and for seminars and presentations.

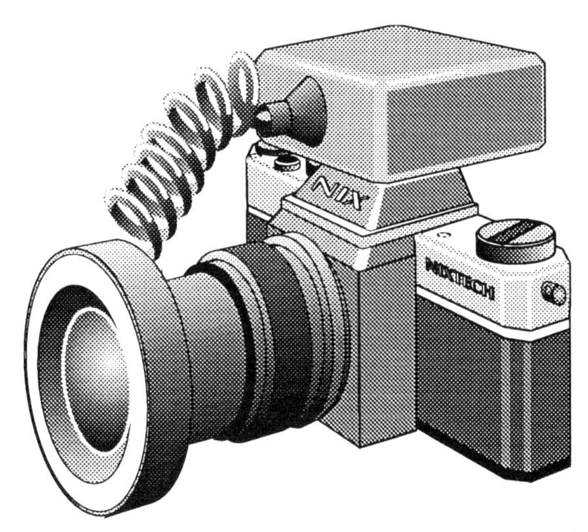

Fig. 92. Dental macro-photography system. 35 mm single lens reflex camera with macro-focusing lens and electronic ring-flash unit.

The mouth presents a number of photographic problems. It is small and therefore magnification is required. It is also dark and difficult to illuminate and so specially-designed lighting is needed. Whilst there are a number of purpose-built dental cameras, most dentists choose to set up their own equipment from the wide range of photographic kit which is on the market today.

A basic kit will consist of a 35 mm single lens reflex camera, a close-up lens and a lens-mounted electronic flash-gun *(Fig. 92)*. Supplementary equipment in the form of cheek or lip retractors and mouth mirrors will also be needed.

Cameras

Single lens reflex cameras *(Fig. 93)* are the best design for clinical photography. Single lens reflex (SLR) means that the camera has only one lens and this is used for viewing the image to be photographed and for taking the picture. In order to achieve this there must be a mechanism whereby the image from the camera can be directed onto the film or through the viewfinder *(Fig. 94)*.

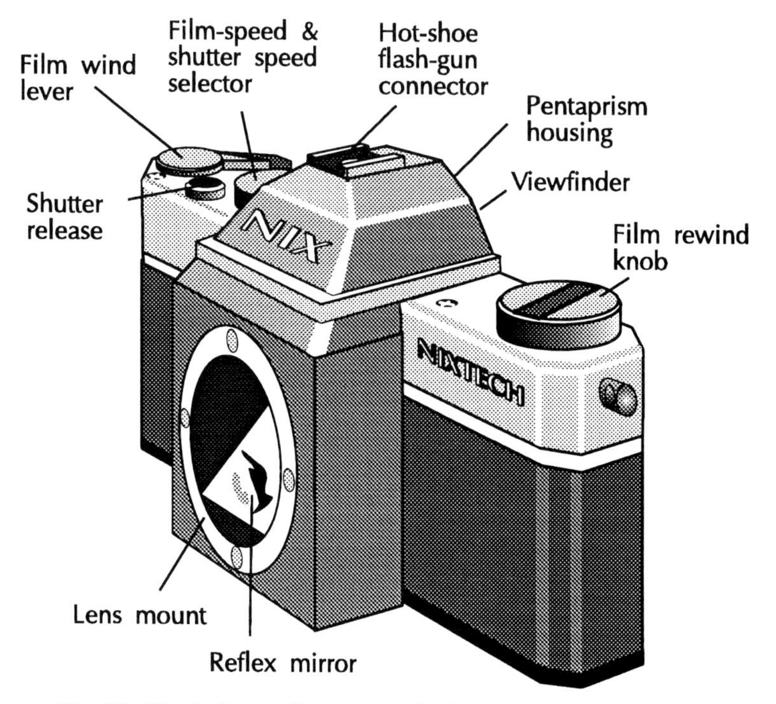

Fig. 93. Single-lens reflex camera body.

A mirror placed in the optical path from the lens to the film intercepts the image and diverts it into a five-sided prism which forms part of the viewfinder. When the shutter release button is pressed the mirror swings up out of the way to clear the path to the film.

No great sophistication is needed in the basic body. Many bodies today are electronically-programmed and are capable of a wide range of function. Dental photography requires only that the shutter should operate accurately at a speed appropriate to that of the flashgun, normally 1/60 of a second. This is not a very demanding requirement by modern standards.

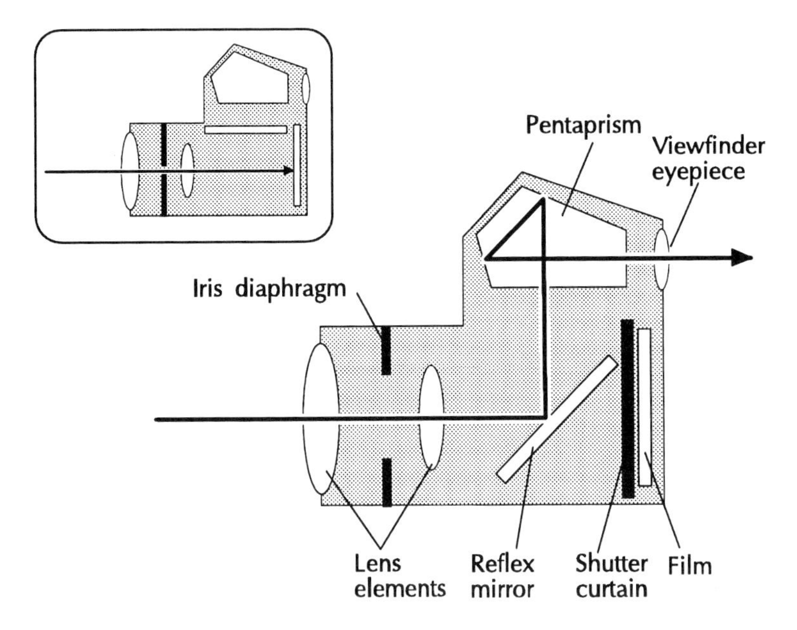

Fig. 94. Light path through SLR camera whilst focusing and (inset) whilst exposing a frame.

One extremely useful function of the camera body is to be able to meter the amount of light hitting the film whilst the photograph is being taken. This information is used to control the electronic flash-gun so that the exposure control is automatic. This is known as through the lens (TTL) flash metering. It is definitely worthwhile paying for this feature because it makes dental photography very much more simple and the results more predictable.

Automatic cameras

Automatic exposure control is a useful feature of a camera system, but in certain circumstances it may be necessary to override it, for example, to take pictures from a computer monitor. Certain camera bodies do not allow this.

Automatic focusing is becoming very common on 35 mm SLR cameras. It can be impossible to operate satisfactorily when the extreme close-up views of dental photography are being taken and is generally best avoided for clinical systems.

The usual film format for clinical photography is 35 mm. This size is universally obtainable and has the greatest range of film choice. The best choice of camera is therefore a 35mm SLR.

Lenses

Lenses *(Fig. 95)* are specified in terms of their focal length, aperture and range of focus. The focal length indicates the angle of view of the lens. A short focal length lens will have a wide angle of view and a long focal length will have a narrow angle of view and act more like a telescope, hence the term 'telephoto lens'. Wide-angle lenses have focal lengths in the range 20–40 mm. Telephoto lenses range from 70–400 mm or above. The middle of the range, 50 mm, is known as a standard lens and has about the same perspective as the human eye. Wide angle lens are useful for landscape photography but have little use in dentistry. For most clinical purposes a medium telephoto lens is most suitable, with a focal length of around 100 mm.

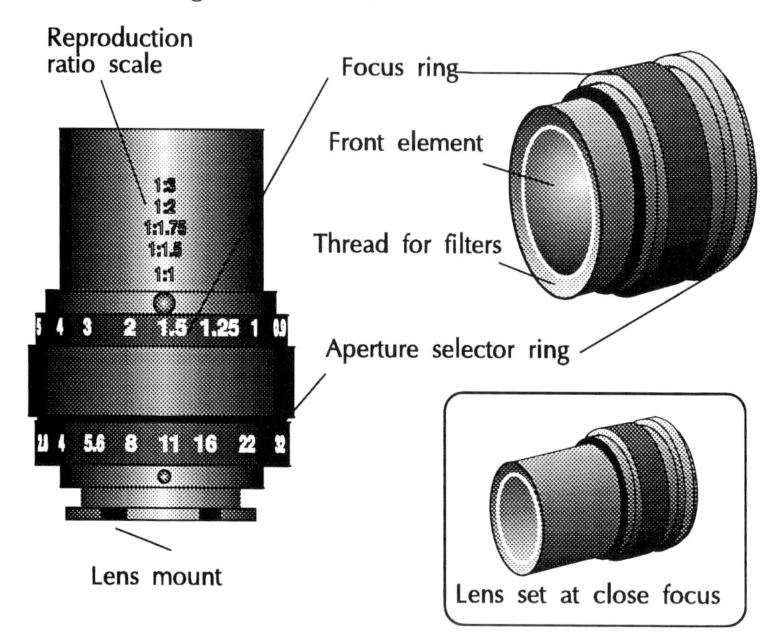

Fig. 95. Macro-focusing lens.

All lenses have a focusing control to enable the lens to focus on subjects at different distances from the camera. Normal lenses do not allow very close focusing but this is an essential for dental photography. The lens must be capable of 'macro-focusing', i.e. focusing on objects which are very close to the lens. This can be achieved by placing a supplementary lens onto the front of the main lens but this arrangement gives a limited range of focus.

Another parameter which specifies a lens is the aperture. Inside a lens there is an iris diaphragm which opens and closes to regulate the amount of light passing through the lens. The aperture is calibrated in 'f stop numbers', ranging f1.2, f1.4, f1.8, f2, f2.8, f5.6, f8, f11, f16, f22, f32. These numbers take into account the inverse square law of light intensity and larger the number, the smaller is the aperture. The stated f number of the lens is the maximum aperture of the lens, the value when the iris diaphragm is wide open and the lens is gaining as much light as it can. The f number will usually be in the range f1.2 to f5.6 depending on the design.

Normally, the aperture is used to limit the light in bright conditions but this function is not needed for dental photography. However, the iris diaphragm has a secondary effect, it alters the depth of focus of the lens. The depth of focus or depth of field is the range of distance over which any object is in clear focus. When the aperture is wide open the depth of field is narrow, when the aperture is closed down the depth of field is greater. In order to focus on the front and the back of the mouth at the same time, or even just to view across a quadrant, a substantial depth of field is required. This means that the lens must be capable of closing down to a narrow aperture, preferably to at least f22 or f32. However, this gives a very dim image indeed and intense lighting is needed to make up for the depth of field, so electronic flash is normally used. But electronic flash cannot be used to illuminate the subject whilst the photographer is composing the image and focusing on the subject. Whilst this is done the iris diaphragm must be opened up to its fullest and a lens with a large aperture is most useful. Closing the aperture down to the setting which has been pre-selected for the photograph is normally an automatic function of modern cameras. The lens used by the author for clinical photography has a focal length of 105 mm and an aperture of f2.8 for focusing which closes down to f32 for taking photographs.

Alternative optics

Close-up rings

Any lens can be converted to close-focusing by the addition of close-up rings. These are hollow tubes which are interposed between the lens and the camera body which enable the camera to focus on objects closer to the lens than the normal adjustment on the lens barrel allows *(Fig. 96).*

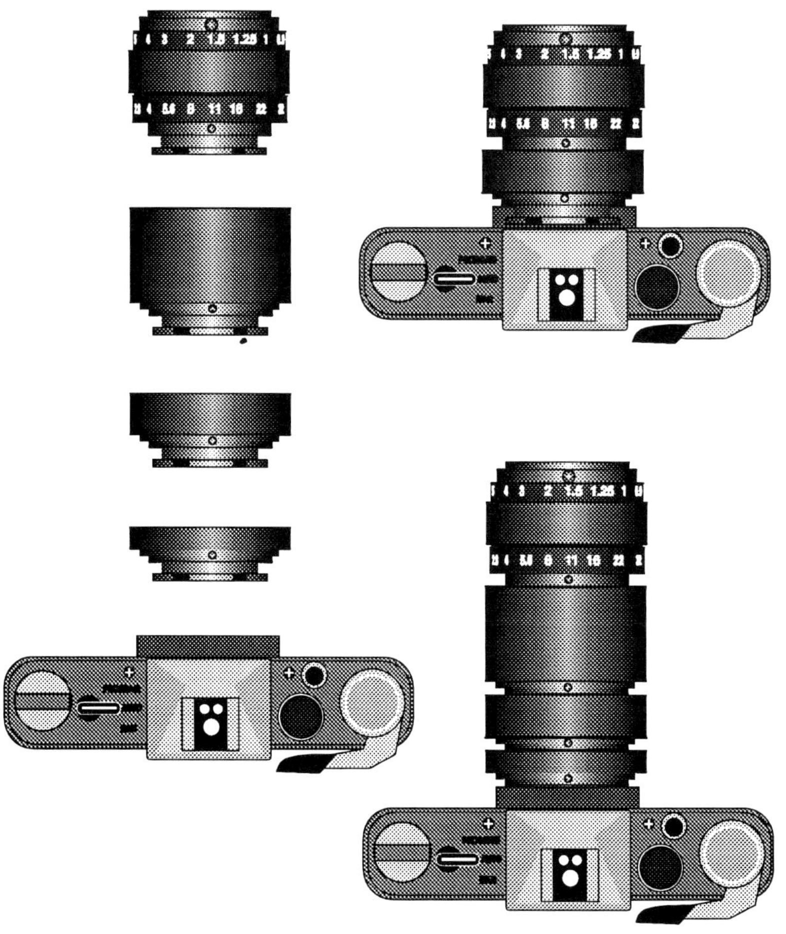

Fig. 96. Close-up rings for macro-focusing with a standard lens.

The tubes are normally sold in sets of three, with a length ratio to each other of 1:2:3. This enables the greatest range of focusing potential. They are cheap but rather inconvenient when compared with a dedicated macro-focusing lens because they require constant reconfiguring to vary the field of view and consequent magnification.

Close-up lenses

Close-up lenses can be fitted to the filter mount of any lens to enable it to focus closer. The strength of the lens is measured in dioptres and a lens of +3 dioptres is the most useful for dental work. Like close-up tubes, they are more restricted in their range of action and can lead to a degraded image. Placing a single close-up lens on the filter mount of a dedicated macro-lens can increase its magnification dramatically for the occasional subject.

Lighting

Lighting for dental photography has two basic requirements. It must be intense and it must be relatively shadow-free. Intensity is needed for reasons dictated by the lens design which are described above. The lighting must be relatively shadow-free so that the subject is illuminated evenly and the lighting is not obstructed by the lips or other tissues, casting shadows over the area to be photographed.

The term 'relatively shadow-free' is chosen with care. Totally shadow-free illumination can be achieved using a coaxial lighting system where the illuminating light beam is projected through the same lens as is used to take the photograph. Such specialist lighting is found in surgical operating microscopes. Totally shadow-free lighting such as this has a major draw-back for dental work. It produces a very flat image with reduced detail of depth and contour. Slight shadowing is desirable so that three-dimensional detail is modelled by the lighting.

Ring-flash units are used commonly in dental photography but they have the disadvantage that they approach shadow-free illumination. The ring-flash consists of an annular flash-tube arranged around the rim of the taking lens and powered from a remote power-supply and control unit *(Fig. 97)*.

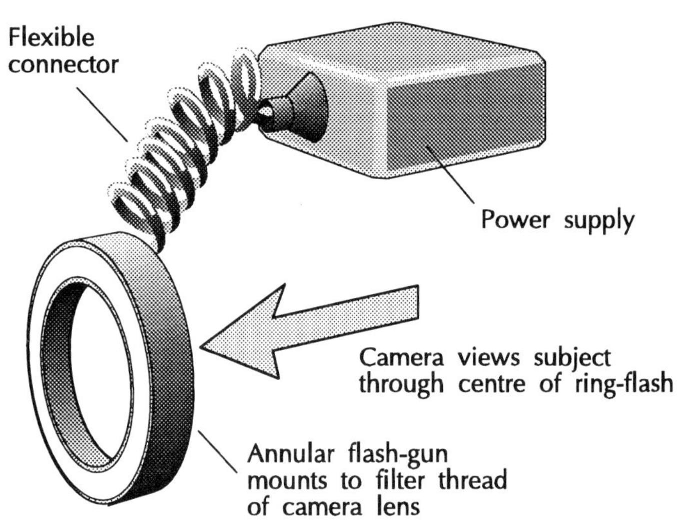

Fig. 97. Ring-flash unit and power supply.

This system is easy to use and acceptable results can nearly always be obtained. However, superior results can be achieved by using one or two point-sources of lighting close to the rim of the lens *(Fig. 98)*. These will model the teeth much better and produce a more dramatic and realistic shot.

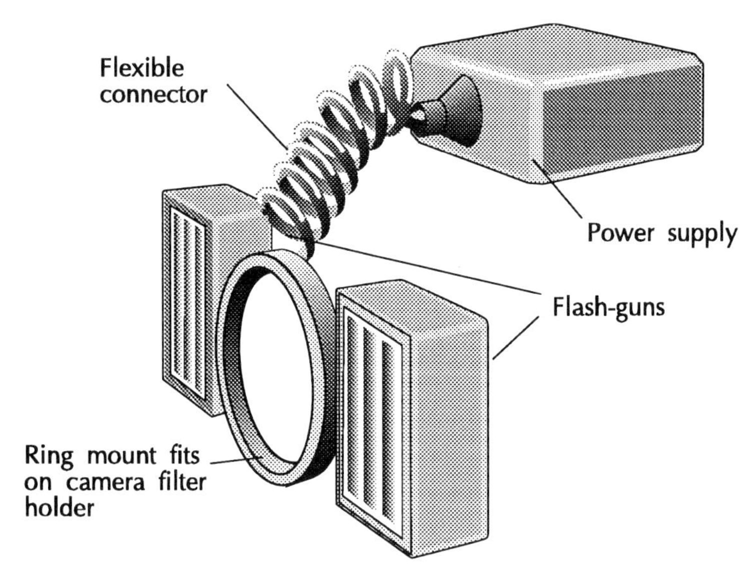

Fig. 98. Twin head macro-flash unit.

Film

Film is available in either colour or monochrome (black-and-white) versions. Monochrome film has little use except for specialist purposes such as publication and so can be disregarded.

There are two types of colour film, negative film for prints and reversal film for transparencies. The choice of film will depend very much on the function of the photographs. Pictures for storage in case-sheets and for patient education are best taken on print film. Pictures for presentation to group audiences need to be recorded on transparency film. Prints can be made relatively easily from transparency film but the reverse is less simple. Therefore if the budget allows it and there is a possiblity of needing the pictures for presentation then it is sensible to use transparency film all the time.

Film is obtainable in a range of speeds. The speed is stated in ASA or ISO numbers and is a measure of the sensitivity of the film to light. There is a balance, the more sensitive the film the less detail it can record. For most clinical photography a speed in the region of 100 ASA is appropriate.

Accessory devices

Photographic mirrors

Good mirrors are usually essential in obtaining a clear view of the area to be photographed. If a standard mirror is used then a double image may be obtained due to light reflecting firstly from the glass surface of the mirror and then from the silver coating on the back of the mirror. This can be avoided by using front-surfaced mirrors. These are manufactured specifically for dental photography and are available from a number of manufacturers. An alternative to front-silvered glass is chromium-plated polished steel. These are easier to clean and can be sterilised more easily, although all photographic mirrors tend to suffer during sterilisation. Photographic mirrors tend to mist up when used intra-orally, but this can be avoided by heating the mirrors to just above body heat prior to use.

Cheek retractors

Cheek retractors are manufactured specifically for dental photography, although the self-retaining retractors used by orthodontists while bonding brackets on will work just as well. It is important to use the retractor correctly and to pull the lips forward as much as possible to gain the best possible view. Metal retractors are not a good idea because they reflect the light of the flash-gun and can flare out the image badly. Transparent plastic retractors work best.

Cross-polarisers

One of the problems with intra-oral photography is that most surfaces to be photographed are wet! This reduces much of the detail which would otherwise be obtained because the illuminating light is reflected back from the surface of the moisture film rather than from the tissue surface underneath.

One method of overcoming this is to use cross-polarising filters, one on the the lens and another on the flash-gun. The filters are set so that they are 90° out of alignment with each other. In this way any light which passes directly from the flash-gun to the lens is blocked by the filter on the lens. Light hitting a non-specular surface, such as soft tissue, is rotated and loses its polarisation. In doing so it becomes visible to the taking lens because it will now pass through the polarising filter on the lens.

This method is very useful for photographing during surgery where irrigants cannot be avoided and soft tissue must be kept wet. It also has use in dermatology for photographing skin where it shows up much of the detail normally hidden by reflection from the surface keratin.

Photographing computer screens

Many programs exist for the creation of text and graphic images for the production of photographic slides. Whilst these are best printed using a dedicated 35 mm optical slide printer, satisfactory results can be obtained by photographing the screen directly. A standard dental macrophotography system will work well if set up correctly. The reader should refer to the section on photographic equipment for more details. The lens should have a focal length around 100 mm and the camera must be mounted on a tripod squarely in front of the screen. The computer monitor should be set to mid-brightness and contrast and the camera set to a shutter speed of one second. The long exposure is necessary because the computer builds up the image on the screen by scanning sequentially horizontal lines down the screen. If too high a shutter speed is used then only part of the image will be recorded. Because the light is being produced by the computer screen and not reflected from it, a flashgun cannot be used. The room should be in total darkness to avoid reflections from the screen.

It will be necessary to expose a test film at various aperture settings to determine the correct values for the particular equipment in use but as a rough guide the aperture should be set to f8 for the first trial shots.

Slide projectors

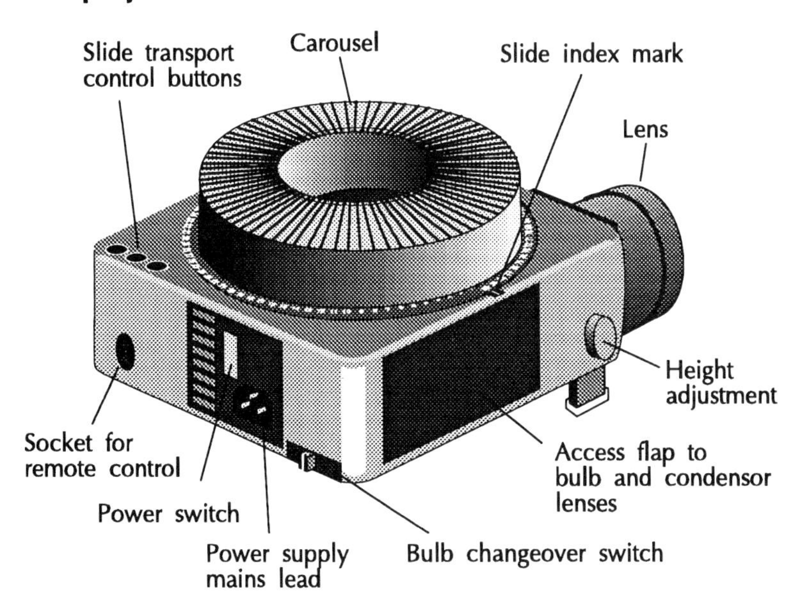

Fig. 99. Outline of the main features of Kodak Carousel slide projectors.

Various designs of slide projector are in use but the most popular system in the UK and USA is the Kodak Carousel projector *(Figs 99 and 100)*. Alternative systems with straight magazines are usually cheaper but many use open trays which spill easily, and usually at the most critical moment when slide magazines are being changed during a presentation.

This system has the advantage that slides can be pre-loaded into magazines which can be sealed closed. This avoids many of the problems of spilt or damaged slides when the cassette is being loaded into the projector.

Slide projectors use tungsten–halogen bulbs as a light source and the majority of colour films are colour balanced so that the colour of the image is correct when projected. For more details of tungsten–halogen bulbs see the section on light activation units (page 13).

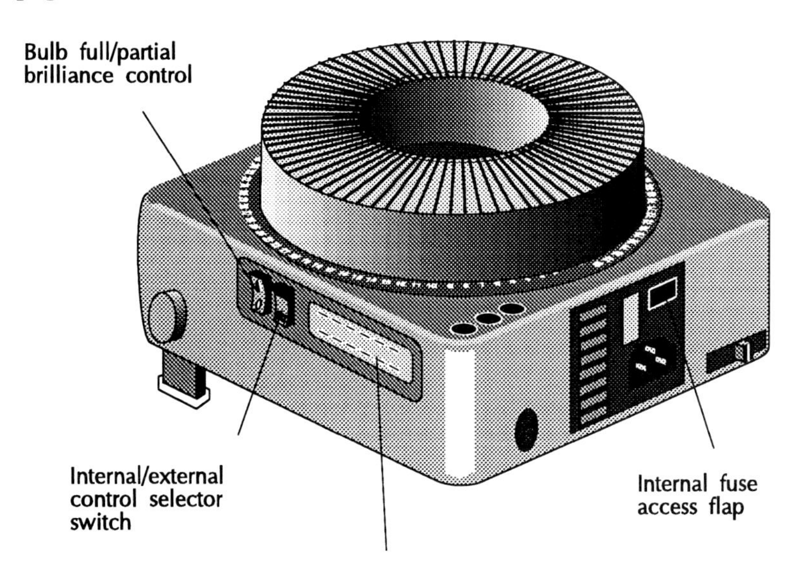

Fig. 100. Outline of external interface on some Carousel projectors.

Slide projectors can be controlled by hard-wired remote controls or by cordless controllers which transmit commands via infra-red transmission. Infra-red systems function very well if set up and operated correctly, but can easily be misused. It is important to ensure a clear line of view between the hand-held transmitter and the receiver at the projector. Some remote links are able to operate by reflection from the projection screen. When this configuration is used the speaker must be instructed to point the remote control to the screen rather than the projector to ensure efficient operation. Whilst infra-red systems can give great freedom of movement to the speaker, hard-wired systems are much more resistant to incorrect configuration.

Quality of image

The brightness of the image is critical to an effective presentation. It is determined by:

1. The size of the projected image.
2. The distance from the projector to the screen.
3. The reflectiveness of the screen which will be determined by the nature of the screen material and its precise colour and surface finish.
4. The aperture of the lens (f or stop number.
5. The condensor system in the projector.
6. The wattage of the projection bulb.
7. The alignment and cleanliness of the optics.

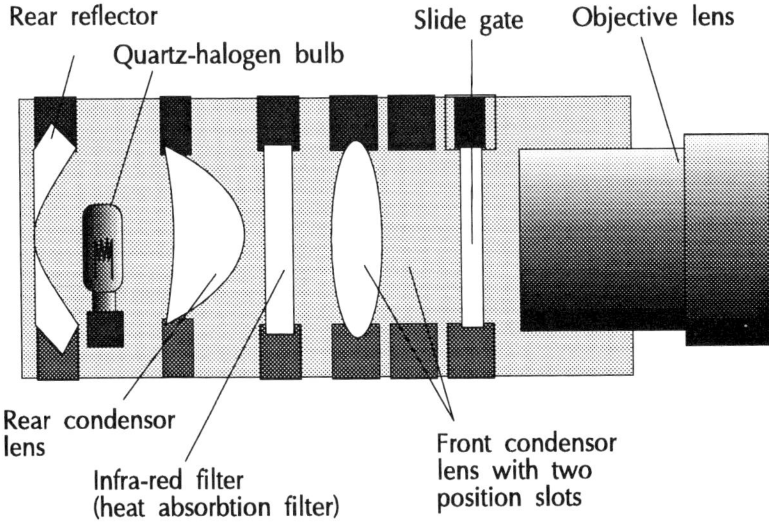

Fig. 101. Optical system in Kodak Carousel projector (accessed through flap in right side).

For maximum brightness of the projected image, the condensor lens system must match the projection lens. Carousel and other projectors have slot-in condensor lens which may be mounted in varying positions depending upon the projection lens in use. This is illustrated in *Fig. 101*. The lens system should be tried out by projecting onto the screen without a slide in the slide-gate. If you are unsure about which slot the condensor lens should be in then it is simple to swap the lens from one slot to the other to determine which image is brightest and illuminates the screen most evenly.

Choice of lens

The focal length of the projection lens determines its field of projection in the same way that the focal length of a camera lens determines its field of view. Zoom lenses are useful but rarely produce the brilliance and linearity of image of a fixed focal length lens. The relationship between the focal length of the lens and the size of the projected image is indicated in *Fig. 102*.

Focal Length of Lens (mm)	Projection Distance (metres)								
	4	6	8	10	12	14	16	18	20
70	1.9	2.9	3.8	4.8	5.8	Possible problems with image brightness			
85	1.7	2.5	3.3	4.1	5.0	5.9			
100	1.4	2.0	2.7	3.4	4.1	4.8	5.5	6.2	
120	1.2	1.7	2.3	2.9	3.5	4.1	4.7	5.3	
150	5.9	1.4	1.8	2.3	2.8	3.2	3.6	4.2	4.6
200	0.7	1.0	1.4	1.8	2.1	2.5	2.8	3.2	3.6
250	0.5	0.8	1.1	1.4	1.7	1.9	2.2	2.5	2.8
	Width of screen image (metres)								

Fig. 102. The relationship between the focal length of the projector lens and the size of the projected image. (Dimensions apply to a standard 35 mm slide projected in horizontal format).

Setting up an auditorium

Ideally, the screens should be set up so that they are clearly visible to each member of the audience above the heads of the people in the row in front. The projectors need to be well out of the way at the back of the room and should be at centre height with the projection screens *(Fig. 103)*. Total black-out is unwise, but lighting should be kept off the projection screen. Custom-designed auditoriums often use 'star-light' tungsten–halogen recessed lighting which projects discretely over the delegates without illuminating the projection screen. Needless to say, at any presentation, exits must be clearly marked and illuminated while the house lights are dimmed.

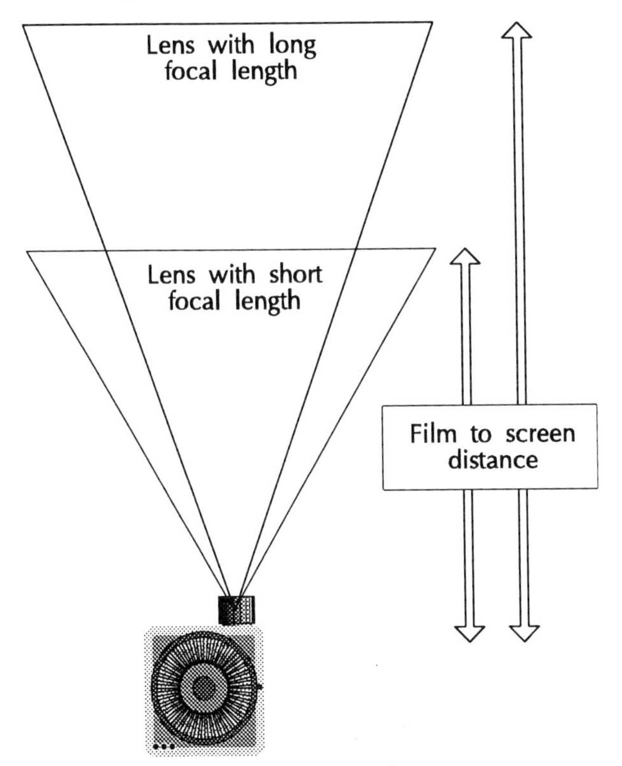

Fig. 103. A short focal length lens is chosen when the projector must be close to the screen. A greater focal length is needed for a larger auditorium.

Sound amplification

The need for voice amplification in an auditorium will vary enormously. The major consideration is the size of the room and the number of people attending. The organisers must not be misled by trying assess the auditorium when it is empty of people because the presence of an audience makes an enormous difference to the acoustics of the room. 50 soft bodies in a room act as significant sound dampers and also provide a background noise which will not be present in the empty room. As a general guide, few speakers will be able to speak at a comfortable volume without amplification to an audience greater than about 30 people.

Sound amplification systems are usually provided in larger auditoriums and require the specialist knowledge of their technicians to be operated optimally. The easiest form of portable sound systems are those built into small desk-top lecterns. These serve the purpose well for the majority of dental meetings.

Laser pointers

A good pointer is essential for many presentations and this is best afforded by a laser unit. Early laser pointers used helium neon gas lasers which consumed batteries at a terrific rate. Modern semi-conductor lasers operate successfully at low voltages and work for many hours continuously on one set of batteries. The mechanism of operation of gas lasers and semi-conductor lasers is described on page 87.

Setting up the projector

Before any presentation the projector should be checked for correct function. The slide transport mechanism should be checked as well as whether or not the bulb operates. If a twin-bulb projector is in use then both the working bulb and the replacement bulb must be tested. Spare bulbs and fuses must always be available together with a small electricians neon screwdriver for checking power supplies and changing the fuses.

Most projectors operate best if they are on the level. Gross tipping of the projector in order to project onto a high screen from a low stand is a recipe for slide jamming. A proper stand matched to the screen is essential for a reliable presentation.

Both the condensor lens system and the projection lens must be clean and dust-free. Lenses can be cleaned with proprietary camera lens cleaning fluids and clothes. Other polishes such as general purpose silicone polishes must not be used.

Preparing slides for presentation

Slides for presentation should be mounted in slide mounts appropriate for the projectors in use. Generally, thin glazed plastic mounts are the most satisfactory because they hold each transparency in the same focal plane. Slide mounts should not be mixed within the batch for the same presentation because varying thicknesses of mounts will cause problems with focusing as the transparencies will not be in exactly the same alignment as each other. Some projectors have auto-focus systems and this will compensate for a slight shift in the film position.

Condensation can be a major problem when slides are transported in luggage between presentations. This problem can be avoided by sealing a bag of silica gel in with the slides to absorb moisture.

All slides in a presentation should be numbered to avoid disaster if they are spilled from a projector tray or confused during loading. It is usual to place a mark on the bottom left of the transparency when it is held so that it is being viewed as it should appear on the screen. The mark will then appear on the top right of the slide when it is rotated and inserted into the slide magazine.

Multiple projector shows

Dual projection

Dual projection refers to the use of two projectors sending their images side-by-side onto two screens or one wide one. For the best effect each projector should be set apart from its partner so that it sits centred on its screen, otherwise considerable distortion can occur. Control of the projectors may be independent or linked depending on the choice of the speaker. Care must be taken to ensure that speakers are aware of the screen configuration;

whether two separate screens are to be used or whether a single wide-screen will allow the adjacent images to merge seamlessly in the centre.

Lap-dissolve

Lap-dissolve projection uses two projectors to project onto a single screen. During slide changes, the image from one projector fades up into the image from the other projector which simultaneously fades down. Slide changing is done in the dark projector ready for the next change. This system avoids the dark interval which occurs during slide changes in a single projector presentation. The seamless fading of one image into another is far less tiring to watch and is very effective visually.

It is essential that identical projectors are used together with identical projection lenses and condensor lenses. Special control equipment is required to operate a lap-dissolve system and the projectors must have appropriate interface sockets to allow connection and operation *(Fig. 100)*.

Storage of photographic materials

Photographic materials require careful storage to maximise their life both before and after exposure. Unexposed films should be stored in a cool dry place. If they are to be stored for a considerable period they should be sealed in an airtight container and frozen in a deep-freeze. Before use they must be carefully and slowly defrosted and allowed to reach room temperature before being unsealed and loaded into the camera. Although theoretically a film is more sensitive to light when it is cooled the possibility of condensation on the film emulsion is a problem.

Colour prints fade gradually if exposed to light. If prints are to be kept on display then they should be placed where they will not be exposed to direct sunlight. Like film stock, prints are best kept cool, dry and in the dark.

Colour transparencies deteriorate markedly with age. They must be kept cool, dry and in the dark if their long-term usefulness is to be maintained. Transparencies which are to be archived can be dried and frozen but great care has to be taken to ensure dry defrosting before they are used.

CHAPTER 12

Compressed Air

Compressed air is one of the most essential services in any dental operatory *(Fig. 104)*. It needs to be delivered with sufficient pressure to drive all the required equipment and in sufficient volume to maintain the pressure.

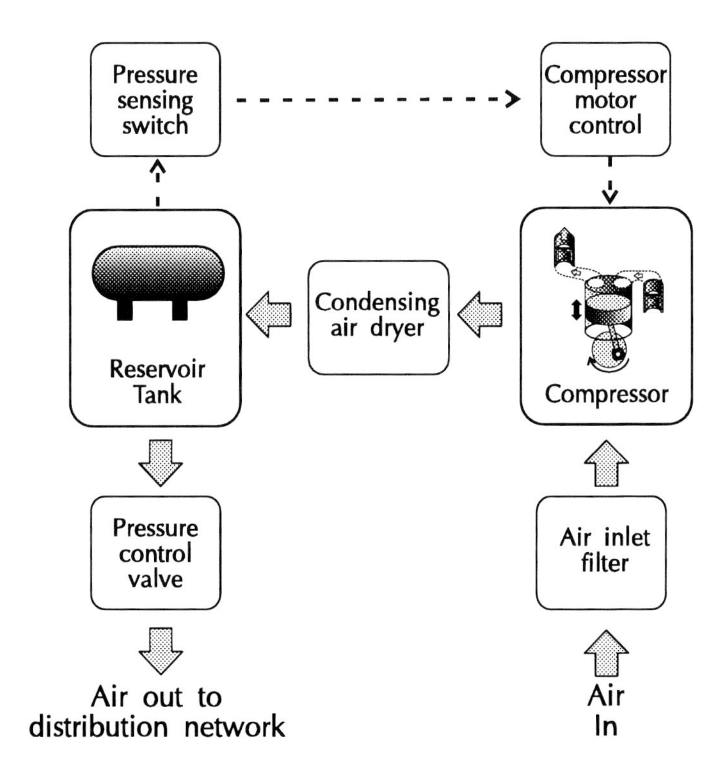

Fig. 104. Dental compressed air system.

The quality of the air delivered is also very important. Compressed air to drive dental equipment needs to be clean and dry. Contamination of the air can occur at several stages between being removed from the atmosphere and delivered to the dental handpiece. Particulate material must be filtered out at the compressor intake and it is sensible to have further filtration along the lines to gather debris shed by the compressing machinery and distributing valves and pipelines. Particulate material forced into the fine-tolerance machinery of dental motors and turbines can cause untold damage. One major source of particulate contamination in a dental school occurred as a result of internal corrosion of the distribution pipes within the building. A design and planning error caused them to be fabricated from iron instead of the more corrosion-resistant copper piping. Extensive filtration has had to be installed and requires intensive maintenance to overcome the problem without installing an entirely new distribution system.

Compressors can be noisy devices and it is sensible to site the compressor as far away from the surgery as possible.

Oil is an inherent component of running machinery and some types of compressor can introduce oil into the air lines. Oil-free compressor stages are available and desirable.

Compressors

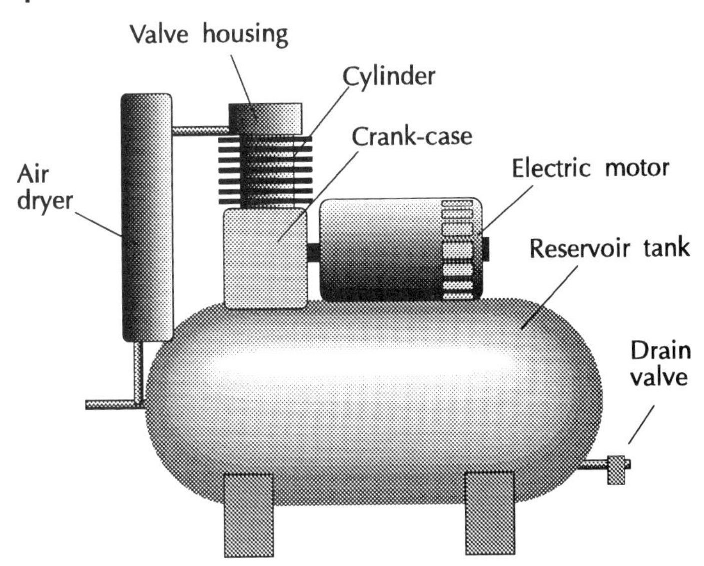

Fig. 105. Dental air compressor.

Compressors *(Fig. 105)* need to provide an adequate flow rate as well as adequate pressure. They need to function with reliability and minimum maintenance. There are three common designs of air compressor; reciprocating piston, rotary vane and diaphragm types.

Reciprocating piston compressor

Reciprocating piston air compressors are the most popular type in use. An electric motor drives a shaft connected to a piston which runs in a cylinder *(Fig. 106)*. Popper valves direct the flow of air in and out of the cylinder as the piston rises and falls. The cylinder head is usually finned to dispose of heat built up during the compression phase.

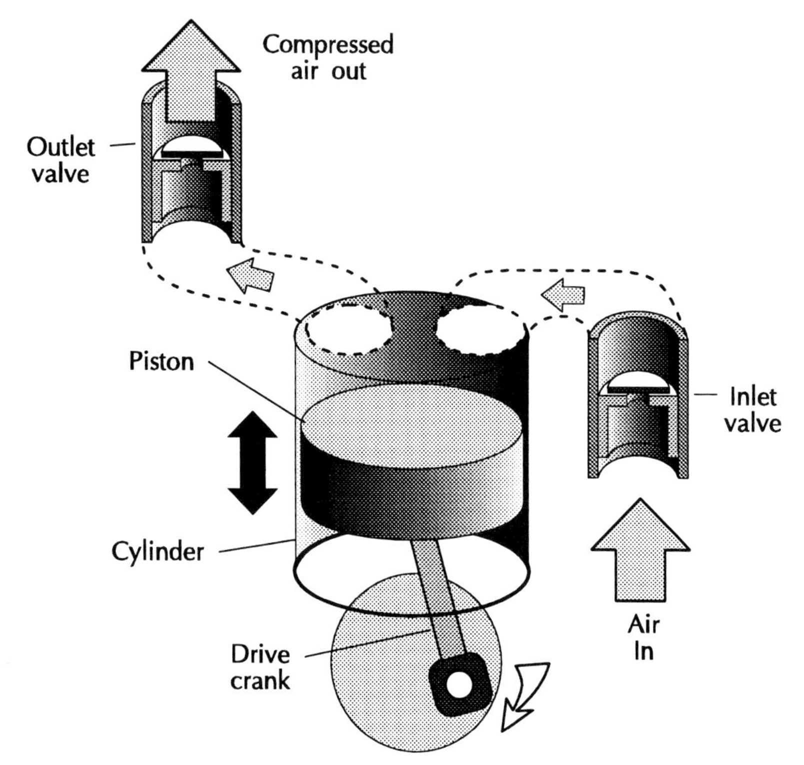

Fig. 106. Reciprocating piston air compressor.

Such compressors can build up considerable pressures but with a lower volume than the rotary vane type which is described below. Several compressors may be driven by a single motor to increase the output volume.

Piston air compressors tend to be the most noisy of all types.

Rotary vane compressor

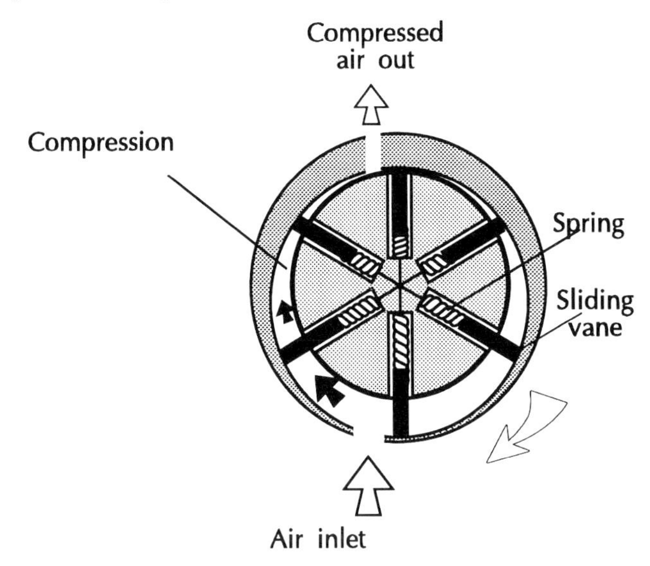

Fig. 107. Rotary vane air compressor.

Rotary vane systems *(Fig. 107)* run quietly and efficiently but the vanes tend to suffer more from wear than the piston type compressors do. The output is constant and smoother than a piston type but there is still some pulsation of pressure as each vane crosses the air outlet aperture. Again, several compressors may be driven by a single motor to increase volume output.

Diaphragm compressors

Diaphragm compressors *(Fig. 108)* are generally clean and reliable though they are not capable of the output pressure and volume of a rotary vane machine. They can be set up in banks feeding a large reservoir tank and in this way the low output rate can be overcome. Diaphragm compressors also have the advantage of being relatively quiet in operation.

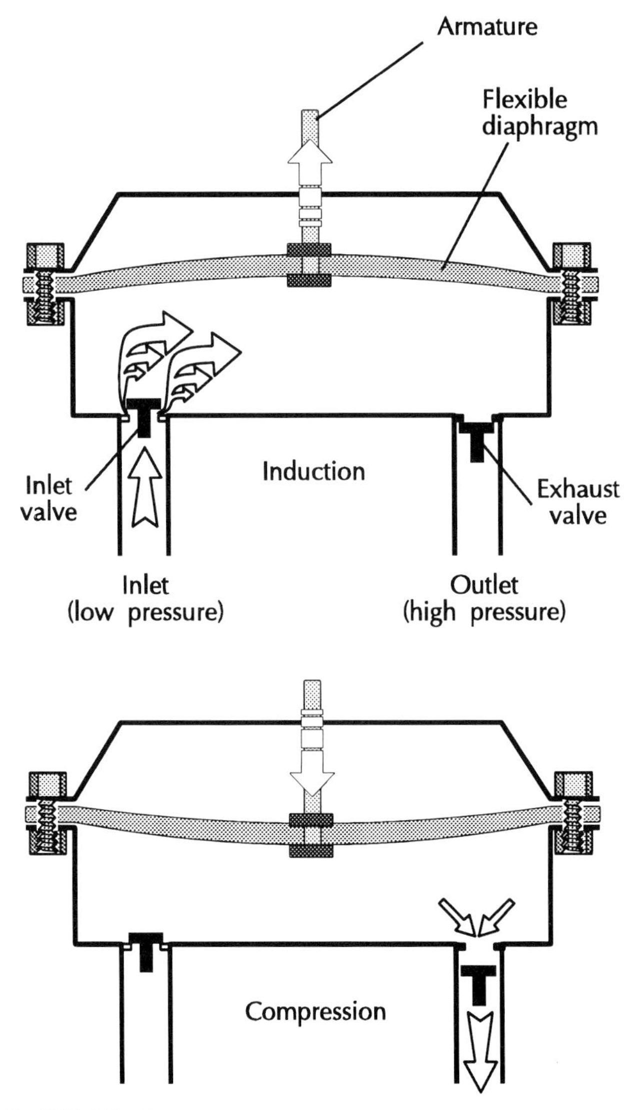

Fig. 108. Diaphragm compressor.

Dryers

As air is compressed it releases heat. For this reason most compressors have cooling fins on the compressor stage. When the air is decompressed it undergoes a reduction in temperature which cause condensation or dew to form. As the air in the receiving reservoir tank is at a lower pressure than the air coming from the compressor, water condenses. Water in the air supply will cause corrosion and contaminate lubricating oils and damage seals if not removed. Compressed air for dental purposes needs, therefore, to be dried before being introduced into the distribution system. Air dryers can be fitted into the air line immediately after the compressor stage and before the reservoir tank.

Reservoir tanks

Control of air pressure within the distribution system is achieved with pressure switches operating the drive motors of the compressors *(Fig. 104)*. A further buffer is required to service large demands on the system over short periods. This is achieved by means of a reservoir tank in the circuit. This is kept compressed at a higher pressure than the distribution network which it feeds by means of a pressure regulator valve *(Fig. 109)*. Reduced pressure in the network opens the valve and the pressure is restored rapidly from the high-pressure reserve in the reservoir tank. When the pressure in the tank falls sufficiently, pressure switches trigger the compressors to replenish the reservoir.

Reservoir tanks may hold a large volume of air under a considerable pressure and require regular inspection and testing to ensure safety. Hydraulic testing to a pressure considerably above the pressure at which safety valves would normally vent ensures that safety is maintained. Such testing must be carried out only by technicians who are trained in such procedures.

As the compressed air from the compressor expands into the reservoir tank it cools, releases water vapour and dew forms. This water accumulates in the bottom of the tank and drain valves are usually installed to allow regular venting of accumulated pools. Regular drainage is important to prevent corrosion in the entire system. Ideally, an air drying stage should be incorporated into the system before the reservoir tank.

Pressure regulators

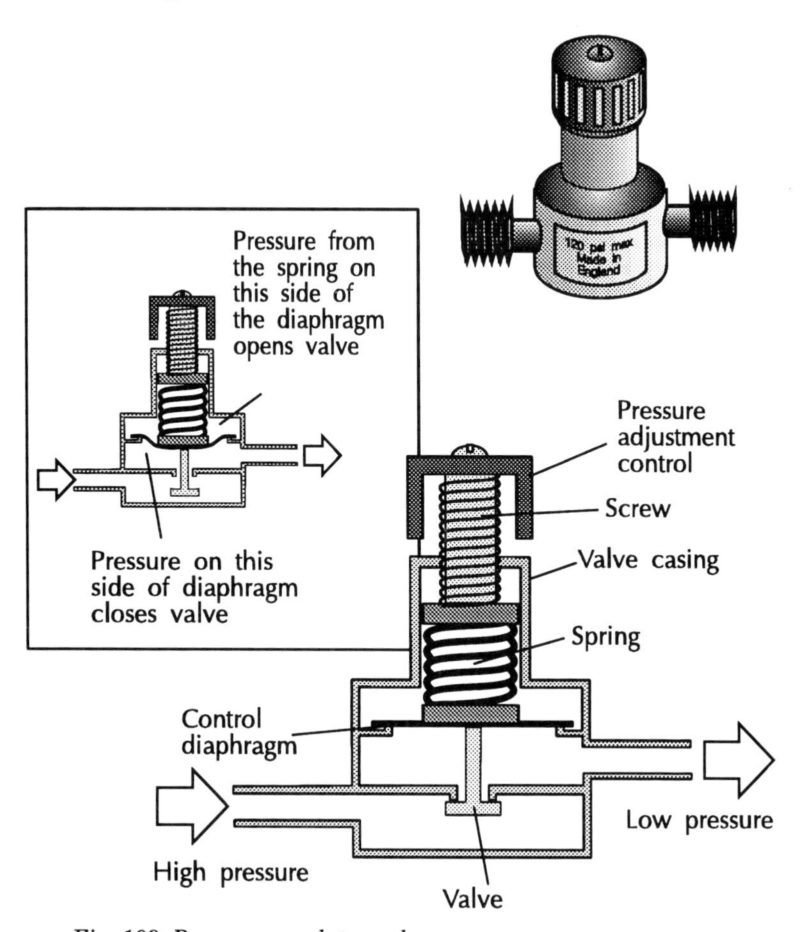

Fig. 109. Pressure regulator valve.

A typical pressure regulator is illustrated in *Fig. 109.* A valve separates the high pressure chamber beneath from the low pressure chamber above. A diaphragm in the low pressure chamber acts on the valve to open or close it. A spring presses against the opposite side of the diaphragm and it is the force of this spring that regulates the pressure in the system. The spring serves to open the valve, pressurising the upper chamber until the chamber pressure on the diaphragm counteracts the spring, lifts the diaphragm and closes the valve. The regulator will control flow only in one direction. An embossed arrow on the side of the regulator body indicates how the device should be incorporated into the circuit.

Pressure regulators such as these will adjust the pressure of liquids and gases. Such regulators form intrinsic parts of all dental units and are found in the compressor circuits, instrument delivery units and the assistant's unit. Miniature versions regulate the pressure of air and water to each individual instrument in the instrument delivery unit including the triple syringe.

Distribution

Compressed air is best distributed through copper piping. This is least susceptible to problems of corrosion and can be formed and joined easily to form a distribution network. The piping needs to be of sufficient diameter to cope with the expected flow rate and volume of air to be delivered. In this respect when designing a distribution system it is far better to allow a good margin for future development and use piping with a larger diameter than is needed immediately. A marginal increase in installation cost may prevent the need to meet the vast cost of a new system at a later date. Compressors can be changed or extra units added with relative ease, repiping a building is another matter.

Control of flow

Compressed air can be switched electrically or mechanically or by compressed air itself. Electric solenoid valves are used commonly and their action is illustrated in *Fig. 110*.

A valve is contained within a non-magnetic casing. It is attached to a magnetic armature which is free to move up and down, operating the valve as it does so. A spring maintains the valve in the closed position by pressing down on the armature. The valve casing is enshrouded by a solenoid coil or electromagnet. When the coil is powered it draws the armature towards its centre against the action of the return spring and in doing so opens the valve. Such valves are directional and usually have an arrow embossed on the side to indicate the line of flow. This is because the pressure on the upper side of the valve assists the return spring in closing it. If the flow is reversed then the valve could be opened against the return spring by the reversed pressure.

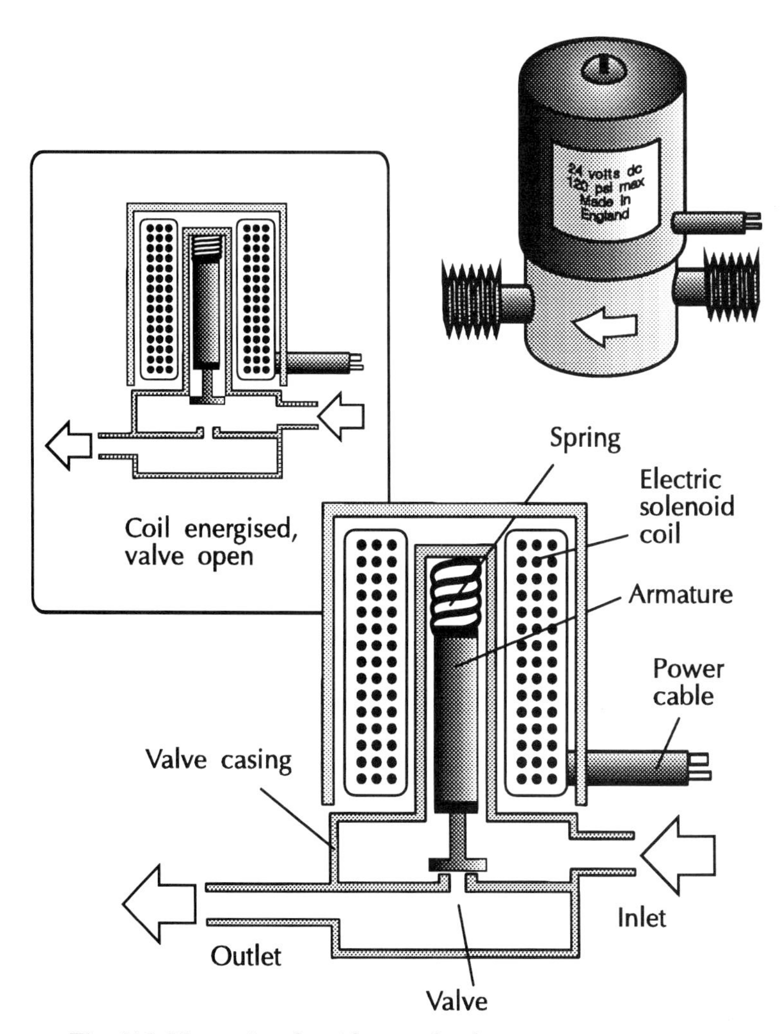

Fig. 110. Magnetic solenoid control valve.

CHAPTER 13

Vacuum Systems

The earliest vacuum systems consisted of a Buchner pump attached to the water supply in the dental unit. This provides a high pressure, low volume suction system and is only useful for removal of saliva from the patient's mouth by means of a tube which is inserted directly into the puddle of saliva. The creation of aerosols from the cooling spray of modern turbines and triple syringes requires a high volume, low pressure suction system for the removal of water.

Early suction systems, or aspirators, built to serve this function were sited in the operatory next to the chair. A centrifugal pump sucked air from the suction hoses through a large bottle. This trapped solids and fluids and the spent air was returned to the surgery. This was less than satisfactory in that the bottle required regular emptying of hazardous waste. Furthermore, the return of contaminated air to the surgery was far from ideal. The trend is now towards centralised suction pumps, remote from the operatory, serving several dental units. Separation and filtration of the aspirate is achieved in a more controlled, and less hazardous, manner.

Vacuum pumps

Various types of vacuum pump exist but for most clinical dental purposes a centrifugal fan type is used commonly *(Fig. 111)*. A helical impeller is mounted in a compression chamber. When the impeller spins, air is blown to the edges of the fan at high speed, creating a powerful vacuum at the centre. Centrifugal fan pumps are used because they provide high volume flow at a relatively low pressure and are very effective at controlling the spray water of the rotary instruments.

Such pumps can be relatively noisy and need to be kept well away from patient flow areas if at all possible.

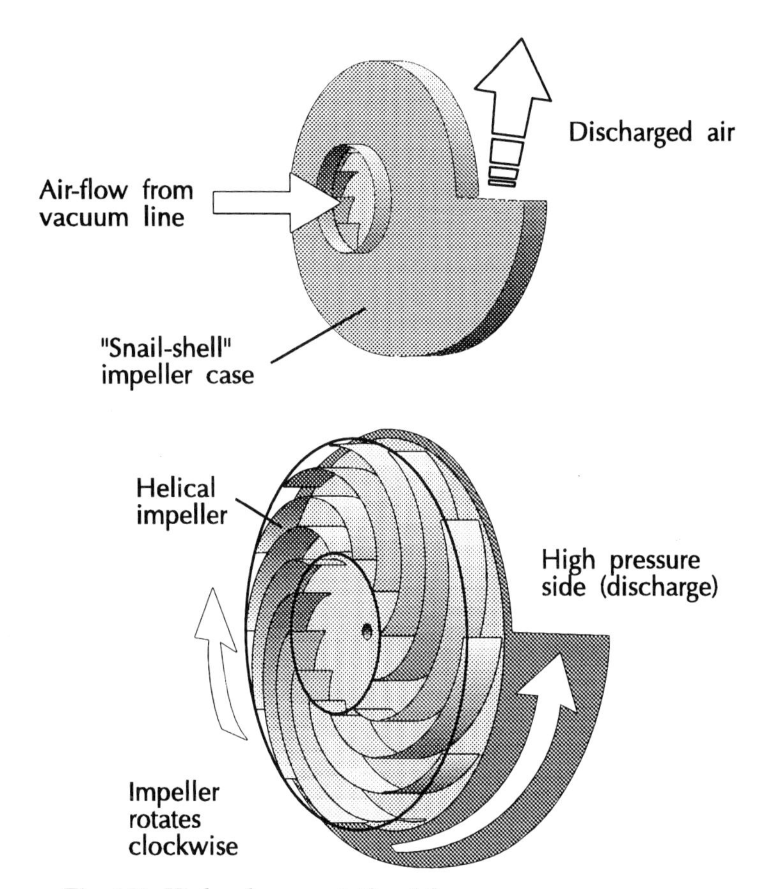

Fig. 111. High volume centrifugal fan vacuum pump.

Distribution

Two main distribution systems exist for suction apparatus, wet-line and dry-line systems. Commonly, wet-line systems are cheaper than dry-line systems because of their greater simplicity.

Wet-line

Wet-line systems separate only solids at the instrument delivery unit or assistants unit in the surgery. Wet air including aspirates is piped to a central vacuum pump and then filtered there, or the wet air is directed into the sewer without separation. Water may be injected into the vacuum circuit to ensure flow and prevent the build-up of debris within the piping.

Dry-line

As the name suggests, dry-line systems use a network of suction pipes which carry air only. Dry-line systems need to separate solids, air and liquids at the dental unit before piping the soiled air to the compressor. The liquids are deposited to the sewers whilst solids are collected in a filter vessel within the unit.

The importance of separation is becoming greater because of regulations preventing the disposal of mercury-contaminated products into the sewer services. Environmental protection cannot allow mercury and heavy metals from dental amalgam to be dumped out of the surgery. Various separator and filter systems now take this aspect into consideration.

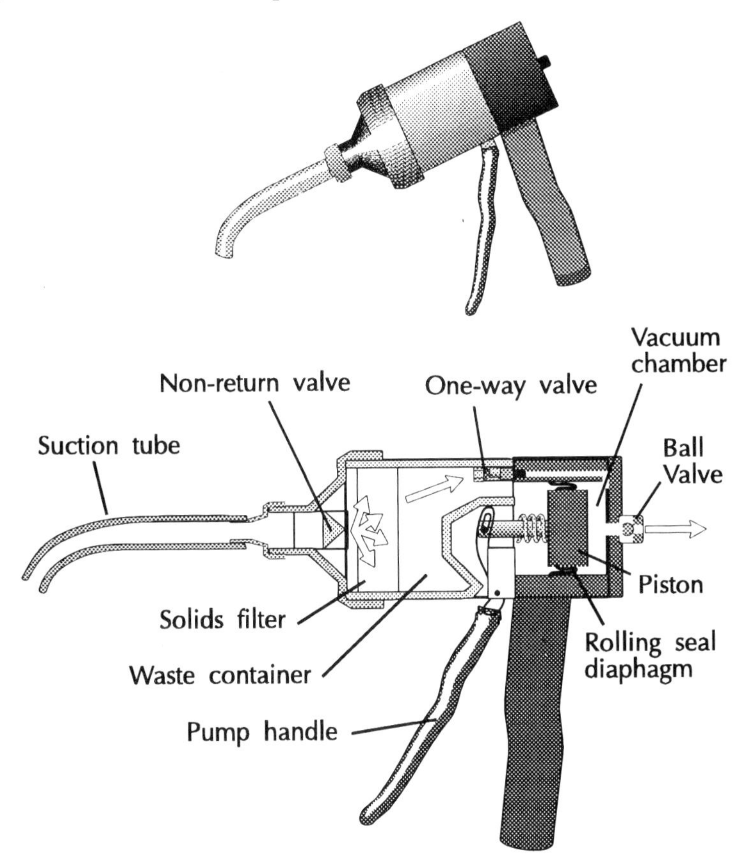

Fig. 112. Hand-operated aspirator.

All vacuum systems require regular flushing with non-foaming detergent cleaners in order to ensure that mechanisms function effectively. The internal components of vacuum systems may be heavily contaminated with hazardous biological material. When such components are being serviced it is important to wear appropriate safety clothing including heavy rubber gloves and eye protection. This is especially true in the case of older units, some of which were not designed with considerations of cross-infection in mind.

Emergency vacuum

Emergency suction should be available for use in resuscitation emergencies. A practical hand-operated pump is illustrated in *Fig. 112*.

CHAPTER 14

Distribution and Piping of Services

Careful design is required to plan appropriate routeing of all the services, especially if they are to be hidden from view but still kept adequately accessible for servicing. False flooring of the type used in many offices and factories seems an obvious answer, but many of these conflict totally with the requirement of having a spill-resistant waterproof flooring which can be disinfected effectively with liquid chemicals.

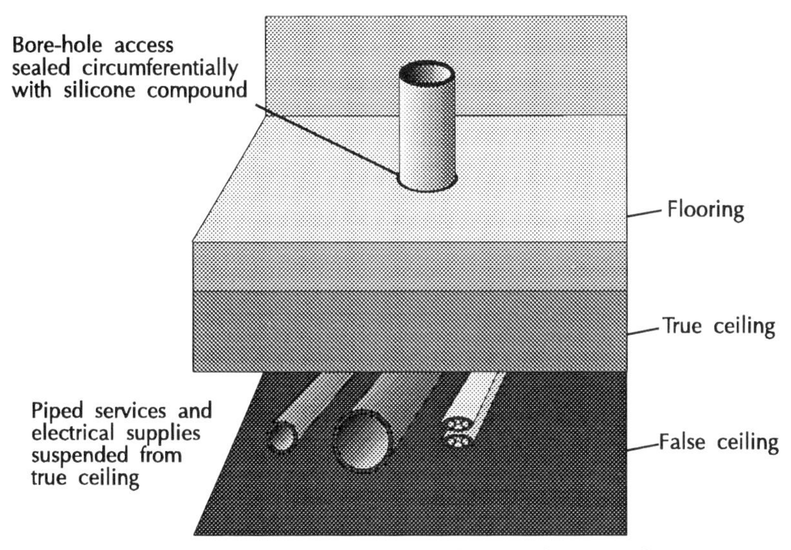

Fig. 113. Services running beneath false ceilings in the room below and delivered to the operatory via sealed bore-holes.

One solution is to have false ceilings in the room below the surgery and to route the services up through bore-holes which can be made water-tight with silicone sealing pastes *(Fig. 113)*. The logistics of such a system are often impossible and compromise is necessary. Modern office buildings are often designed with a perimetric channel at the base of structural walls which carry the necessary services *(Fig. 114)*.

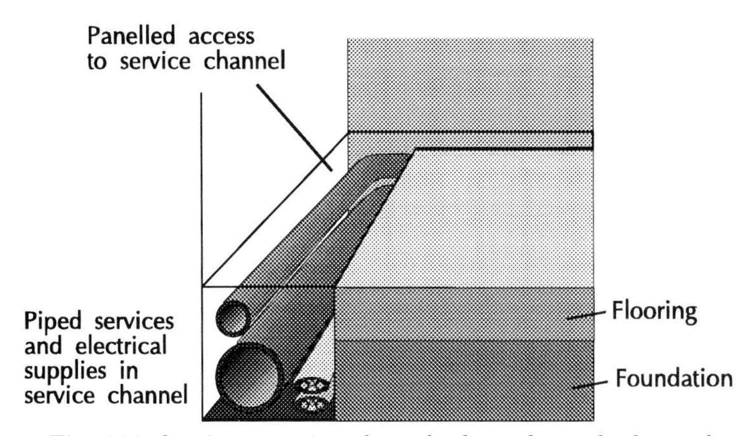

Fig. 114. Services running through channels at the base of structural walls.

Electrical Systems

Electrical safety

Electrical safety is of paramount importance in all equipment used in, or in association with, the treatment of patients. Electrical safety regulations differ between countries and will depend on the conventions which have been adopted for wiring circuits. In the UK, all electrical items are protected from overload damage by a fuse of the correct rating incorporated into the plug. This is not implemented in Continental European and American systems and alternative methods are used. All UK plugs are earthed, whereas two-wire unearthed supplies are still found in the rest of Europe where earth-leakage circuit-breakers are more common.

Professional advice from certified electricians who are aware of local safety requirements for industrial wiring is essential in ensuring safe operation and compliance with local regulations.

Low voltage systems

Voltages in the region of 12–24 volts do not create an electric shock hazard under most circumstances. For this reason the vast majority of dental equipment operates on low voltage provided by an isolating, voltage-reducing transformer.

Isolation transformers

The danger of electric shock in mains-operated equipment can be reduced by isolating the system from earth using an isolating transformer. In this way it is necessary for the victim to touch both wires of the circuit to suffer an electrical shock. Contact with one wire alone will not lead to a shock even if the victim is earthed. This method can be used to isolate older equipment which does not use low-voltage sub-circuits in parts of the system which may present a hazard to the patient. Some older dental units used full mains-voltages in the control switches on the chair-back in solenoid valves used to switch air and water to handpieces.

Earthing

Effective electrical earthing is necessary for many items of equipment. At the time of installation of such equipment it is important to ensure that the electrical supply to the building is provided with an effective earth. Many older buildings have an inadequate earthing system with a wire tied to a spare water pipe or similar.

Earth-leakage safety breakers

All mains-powered apparatus which may come into contact with the patient or dental personnel should be protected with an earth-leakage safety breaker. This device detects the relative flow of current through the live and neutral wires of the circuit. If a leak to earth occurs then the current is shut off immediately. Fast-acting electronic circuitry is used so that the victim is not exposed to an electric shock long enough to be injured.

CHAPTER 15

Environmental Control

The working environment

Environmental control must ensure an adequate air temperature is maintained. To ensure patient comfort this is best kept at a level well above the usual office minimum. Conservation of energy dictates that heat should be preserved within the room, but this may conflict with the need to ensure adequate ventilation. Chemical vapours are unavoidable in the operatory and these must be kept to a minimum. Such contaminants will include mercury vapour, volatile solvents in dentine-bonding agents, vapours from cleaning fluids, etc. Specific provision should be made for air-scavenging if anaesthetic gases are used in any form.

Quality of air

The air in the dental operatory should be changed frequently, well above the rate which would be normal for a contemporary office environment. Forced ventilation to allow rapid air change should be possible after significant releases of air-borne chemicals have occurred. This may happen after swabbing down the work-surfaces with disinfectants or after accidental spillages of volatile chemicals. It is also essential for the rare occasion when a patient may vomit!

The specific requirements of environmental control in a dental operatory should be taken into account at the design stage. Commissioned architects and designers should be made aware of this aspect when plans are being draw up. Significant problems may occur however, when a dentist is using premises which have been designed for other purposes. In many cases the problem can be addressed by simply opening a window, but in air-conditioned office buildings this may not be possible. If a single air-conditioning system maintains the whole building, then the dental practice may encounter massive difficulties in addressing this problem.

Ventilation

Ventilation of a room may be either passive or active. A dental operatory requires both. A simple electrical fan let into an outside window is the minimum requirement for active ventilation.

De-humidifiers

The humidity of a dental operatory may vary considerably and may require active control. Dryness of the air is less of a problem than dampness because of the nature of the equipment and procedures which take place. One of the greatest causes of excessive humidity is the surgery autoclave. More sophisticated models vent externally but simpler ones release a distinct puff of vapour every time the door is opened to remove the instruments. This can cause a significant problem with condensation within the building. Other sources of humidity include aerosols from air turbines, ultrasonic scalers and by evaporation from surfaces which have been swabbed down with disinfectants and are drying out.

Whilst active ventilation may deal with most problems, de-humidification may be necessary especially in more humid climates.

De-humidifiers are generally cheaper to purchase and operate than full air-conditioning units. They have a cooling circuit which causes condensation of atmospheric moisture by cooling the air, and a heat exchanger which returns the heat to the air prior to discharge back into the room.

Air conditioning

Air-conditioners can improve the comfort of surgery personnel and patients enormously. In some countries they are absolutely essential and are taken for granted. However, in other climates they can also be used to great benefit. A good air-conditioning unit should clean the air, remove pollutants and adjust the temperature and humidity to comfortable levels. It should operate silently and effectively, creating no draughts and operating without any irritation to personnel. It should require low-maintenance and should be of a clean design which will not build up its own flora of bacterial or fungal contaminants.

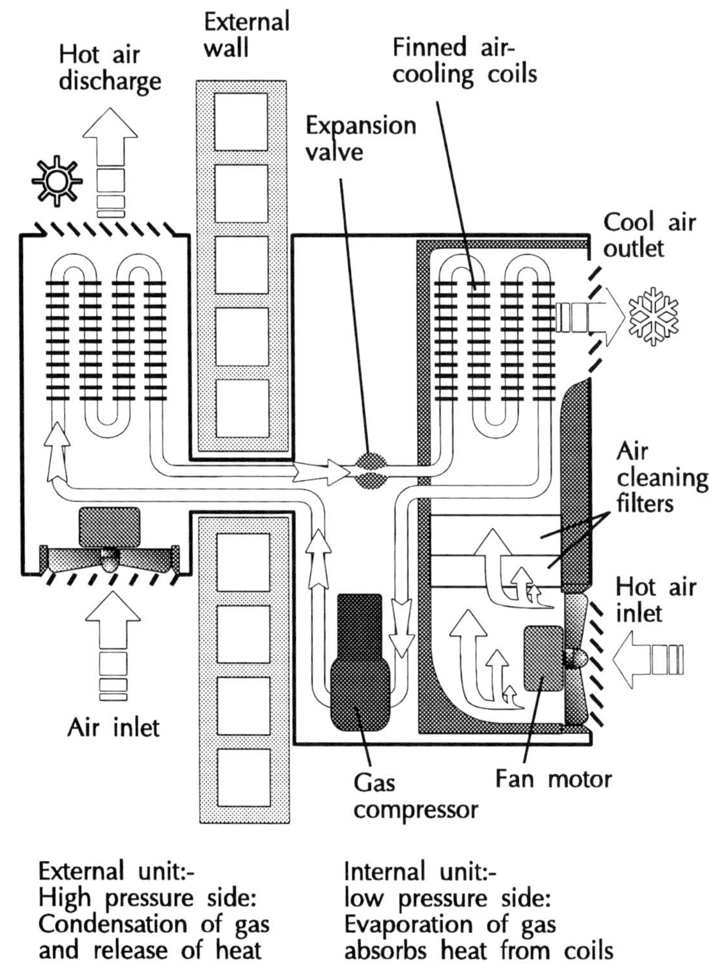

Fig. 115. Small single-room air-conditioning unit.

Small single-room air conditioning units are suitable for most dental practices. Such an installation is illustrated in *Fig. 115.*

Room air is drawn into the unit by an electric fan and passed through a number of air-cleaning filters. The air then passes across a series of finned pipes which cool it before it is returned to the room. The cooling pipes are part of a gas circuit which is the same as that found in a domestic refrigerator. A gas is compressed by an electrical compressor causing it to condense and lose heat. During this phase it passes through an external radiator outside the building and the heat is lost to the atmosphere. The cooled liquid then passes back into the building and through a narrow nozzle or expansion valve leading into a zone of low pressure. As the gas expands into the low pressure cooling coils it absorbs heat from the surrounding room air through the metal of the fins and pipe-work. This gas then re-enters the compressor and passes outside the building to lose this heat in the condensor system once again.

Such units are used for air cooling rather than heating although electrical heating elements are installed in some models. Winter-time heating is best looked after by the building heating system.

Legal aspects

In most countries it is the legal duty of employers to ensure a comfortable working environment for their employees. Dentists, as employers, should make themselves aware of the local and national law in this respect and ensure that all areas of their practice environment, from the waiting areas to the laboratories, comply with such regulations.

CHAPTER 16

Sterilisation Equipment

Autoclave

The autoclave is the best method of sterilisation of dental instrumentation. The instrument pack is heated in steam under pressure until conditions are reached which are beyond the survival capacity of any micro-organism.

An autoclave consists of a chamber which can be filled with steam under pressure. The chamber can be opened to insert and remove the load to be sterilised and then sealed easily to hold in the pressurized steam *(Fig. 116)*.

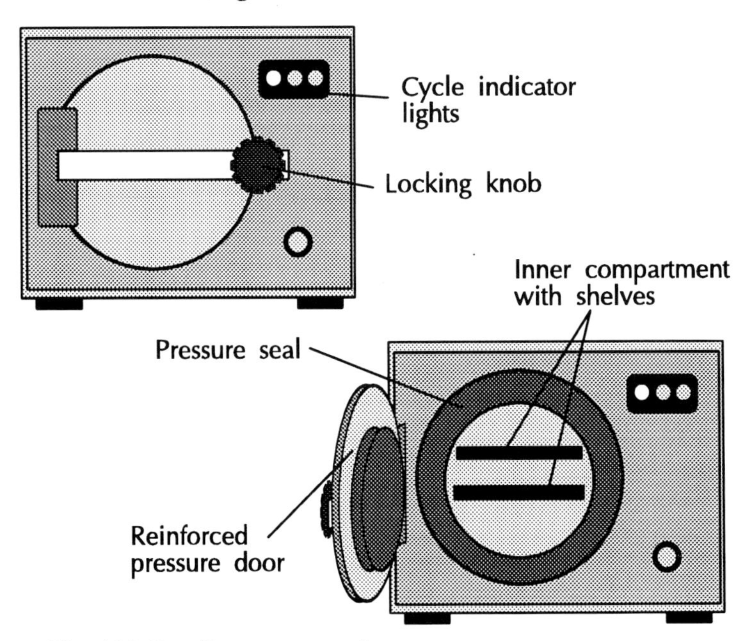

Fig. 116. Small surgery autoclave.

An autoclave must reach and sustain a temperature of 121°C for 15 minutes or 134°C for 4 minutes in order to guarantee sterilisation.

A full-size autoclave suitable for installation in a hospital is a sophisticated piece of machinery. After the sterilisation cycle is complete the autoclave chamber is evacuated in order to remove all traces of water vapour. A dry load is delivered from the machine.

Small simple autoclaves are categorised by the British Standards Institution as 'Transportable steam sterilisers'. After sterilising the load, these cool and condense the steam as water within the sterilisation chamber. More sophisticated models dry the instrument trays off by electric heating.

Modern autoclaves use electronic programming and monitoring of the conditions established in the steam chamber in order to ensure that sterilisation is achieved.

Hot-air steriliser

Hot-air sterilisers are an acceptable alternative to the autoclave. Hot dry air sterilises effectively but takes longer than wet heat. Hot air sterilisers are basically simple electric ovens. The best models have a timer and a door interlock switch to ensure that the conditions for sterilisation are achieved.

Chemical autoclaves

Formaldehyde–alcohol vapour pressure steriliser is the correct name for what is often referred to as the chemical autoclave. The advantages of this system are that instruments do not corrode, the load is dry after sterilisation and the cycle is relatively fast. The process creates a vapour by heating a deodorized alcohol–formaldehyde solution to 132°C at 0.15–0.3 Megapascals for 20 minutes. During the cycle the pre-heated vapour condenses on the instruments. The system is excellent in maintaining the working life of instruments for it does not corrode nor heat-damage the surface of metals. However, the safety of formaldehyde vapour is questionable and for this reason the machines are not in wide use.

Other systems

There are no technologies other than the autoclave and the hot-air oven which have very much use in sterilising dental instruments. Alternative systems are either ineffective or are prohibitively expensive.

Hot water sterilisers

Hot water 'steriliser' is a total misnomer. Hot water sterilisers are inefficient and may be a source of cross-contamination of instruments. Few such sterilisers reach an adequate temperature to destroy spores. These devices have no place in dentistry today.

Glass bead sterilisers

The glass bead steriliser has a role limited to disinfecting endodontic instruments during use. A small ceramic pot is filled with fine glass beads and heated electrically. Endodontic instruments can be inserted amidst the glass beads which conduct heat to the instrument and disinfect the surface. The device does not sterilise reliably and the handles of the instruments remain contaminated. A further problem is that beads of glass may become stuck to the instrument surface and may be transferred to the root canal. To avoid this possibility and to make spills easier to clear up the glass beads can be replaced with common salt.

Chemical systems

The only effective cold chemical sterilising system is activated glutaraldehyde. Instruments are placed in a bath of the solution and left for an appropriate period, usually in excess of 8 hours. In order for the solution to operate it must reach all surfaces of the instruments to be sterilised. Air trapped in crevices or in voids will protect micro-organisms from contact with the solution. Accretions of dirt and organic contaminants must be washed off the instrument before immersion for similar reasons.

Soaking metals in such solutions results in corrosion if steps are not taken to prevent it. Anti-corrosion buffering agents can be added to the glutaraldehyde solution to reduce metal corrosion.

Filter sterilisers; micropore systems

Filters are sometimes introduced into water lines to remove bacteria. In this respect they can be quite effective but viruses still get through. Flow through micropore bacterial filters is very limited.

Specific sterilisation problems

Elevators

Elevators need special care because of the construction of the handle. Often, the handle is hollow but sealed. Heating it in certain high temperature sterilising systems can cause the gas trapped inside the handle to burst it in an explosive manner. Most elevators can be autoclaved safely because of the increase in ambient pressure which accompanies the heat of an autoclave.

Hand instruments

Most hand instruments are relatively easy to clean and sterilise. Scalers and chisels require the additional step of sharpening or honing. Abrasive stones can be used to sharpen steel instruments.

Forceps and orthodontic pliers

Forceps and orthodontic pliers have the added complication of a hinge which may seize if the instrument is sterilised inappropriately. After thorough cleansing of the instrument prior to sterilisation, the hinge should be lubricated with a suitable heat-resistant silicone oil. Care must be taken in ensuring that an appropriate oil is used because some oils deteriorate in the steam cycle of the autoclave and can gum up the hinge mechanism.

Handpieces

Inappropriate sterilisation procedures can and do reduce the life of dental handpieces very considerably. In principle, effective regular cleaning and lubrication should help to prolong the life of a handpiece, but this is not always achieved. Prior to sterilisation handpieces must be cleansed thoroughly and lubricated with an oil approved by the manufacturer.

Storage of instruments

Instruments need to be stored appropriately to maintain sterility and prevent corrosion. A dry atmosphere is essential. Anti-corrosion vapour paper can be placed in drawers with instruments to help protect them. Instruments which have been through inappropriate sterilisation or have been dried inadequately after removal from the autoclave are likely to have their useful service life greatly reduced.

Space disinfection

Large space disinfection of the operatory area is difficult to achieve. Chemical wash-downs of working surfaces should be performed regularly to maintain hygiene. Floors should be designed so that dirt is not trapped. Ideally, the surface should be sealed and the edges and corners of the flooring rounded up into the skirting. The floor of the operatory should be cleansible with liquid disinfectants containing hypochlorite.

Ultraviolet lighting

Ultraviolet lighting can provide some level of large space disinfection. An ultraviolet lighting system can be installed in the operatory and activated when the operatory is in disuse at night. It is important to consider that the effect of such systems is adjunctive only and no effect will occur in areas which are not illuminated directly. Electrical interlocking with the operatory door is sensible to avoid accidental exposure of personnel to ultra-violet radiation.

Some instrument storage cabinets in contemporary dental units are fitted with ultraviolet lights to help maintain clean conditions. The value of these is limited but they will help to reduce contamination on the surface of instrument bags. It is important to recognise that these cabinets are useful only when instruments are sterilised and sealed in suitable containers before being stored in the cabinet.

CHAPTER 17

The Dental Laboratory

Furnaces

Pre-casting

Casting is one of the commonest procedures undertaken in the dental laboratory. Many dental restorations ranging from metal crowns through to partial denture frameworks are made by the lost-wax process. The lost-wax process of casting metals consists of immersing a pattern in a high melting point investment and then burning the pattern out after the investment has set. This creates a void which is the shape of the pattern and into which the casting alloy is forced. The burning out process is accomplished in an electrically-heated or gas-fired furnace. This stage is completed immediately prior to casting so that the investment is at a high temperature when the molten metal alloy is cast into it. This is necessary in order to prevent the alloy shock-freezing and creating an incomplete casting.

The furnace consists of a metal chamber which is lined with heat-resistant ceramic blocks. The muffle is heated by either electrical resistance heating coils or gas flames. A ventilation system is necessary to remove the fumes from the patterns which are, literally, burnt out of the investment rings.

Electrical furnaces consume a considerable amount of power and usually require a special electricity supply to be installed. Some versions use a higher voltage than standard (415 volts in the UK).

Casting

The wax is burnt out in the pre-casting furnace leaving a void which has the shape of the component to be cast. Molten metal is then forced into the void to form the metal casting. Various methods of melting the metal and of forcing into the mould are available.

The simplest method of melting metal is with a gas–air torch. Gas is mixed with compressed air and burnt. The technician selects a reducing atmosphere by placing the reducing part of the flame over the alloy during melting. Oxidation of the metal during the melt-down is limited in consequence.

Electrical methods of melting are available. A plasma arc can be created electrically and used to melt metal. This is quick but oxidises the metal and can easily overheat the alloy if not used appropriately.

The most sophisticated way of melting it is to do so by electrical induction. An alternating current is passed through a coil which surrounds the metal in a ceramic crucible. This creates an alternating magnetic field in the metal ingots. Eddy currents are induced in the metal by this field and these generate heat sufficient to melt the alloy. The vessel in which this takes place can be flooded with an inert gas to ensure that the oxidation of the metal during melting is avoided. This system produces extremely clean castings.

Vacuum furnaces

The sintering of porcelain to construct aesthetic porcelain restorations and porcelain-bonded-to-metal restorations requires high temperatures and reduced pressures. These conditions are provided by vacuum furnaces *(Fig. 117)*. The heart of the furnace is the muffle. This is a cylinder of heat-resistant ceramic which is lined with the coiled coils of an electrical heating element. A porcelain-firing furnace should be capable of reaching a maximum temperature in the region of 1200°C. In the vacuum furnace this lies within a metal chamber which can be sealed from the atmosphere and evacuated by a vacuum pump.

To achieve the working temperature, most furnaces consume around 1.5 kilowatts of energy. This is an intermittant load and will be switched by the controlling thermostat. This amount of energy can be provided by a standard domestic ring main and does not require special electrical wiring to be installed for individual furnaces. However, if multiple furnaces are to be used simultaneously at the same site then special wiring may be necessary to cope with the increased load, especially while the furnaces are heating up to the working temperature.

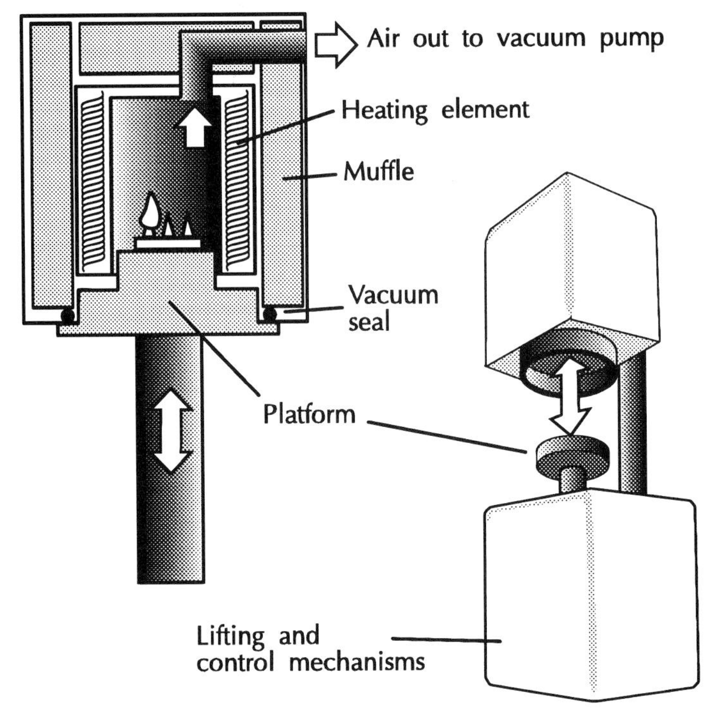

Fig. 117. Vacuum furnace for porcelain.

Modern furnaces vary in design and level of sophistication. A popular design is to have the work elevated into the furnace from underneath by a rising platform, the mechanism of which may be powered and automated. The most sophisticated models are operated by a microprocessor with programmable memory. This microcomputer monitors conditions inside the furnace with temperature and pressure sensors and operates the movement of the work in and out of the furnace with electrical actuators. A range of programs can be stored on removable battery-backed RAM memory cards.

Soldering

Soldering is the joining of two pieces of metal by melting an alloy of lower melting point between them. Soldering is used in orthodontics to join metal components in orthodontic appliances and in bridge-work to join components of bridges which have been cast separately. Soldering irons of the type used in electronics are of little value in dentistry because the tin-lead alloy has inadequate strength for any useful purpose.

Stainless-steel can be soldered using silver solder. The melting point of silver solder requires a considerable heat source to be used. Direct use of a gas–air flame is adequate but the best device is the hydrogen–oxygen generating cell. This device breaks down water electrolytically to produce hydrogen and oxygen. These are fed through a fine needle-shaped nozzle and then burnt to create a tiny flame of very high temperature.

Welding

Welding is the joining of two pieces of metal by melting their surfaces to fuse them together. Sometimes a third metal is fused between the two metals to be joined.

The most common use of welding in dentistry is in orthodontics. Orthodontic welders are electrical resistance welders and do not use a welding metal between the surfaces to be joined. Electrical resistance welding works by clamping the two pieces of metal to be joined tightly together and then passing a low-voltage, high amperage electrical current through the interface. The high resistance of the metals where they are pressed together causes the local generation of considerable heat which melts the two surfaces. The pressure forces the molten surfaces together and a strong bond is formed.

Spark erosion

Spark erosion is a method used extensively in the engineering industry for making precision metal components. An accurately constructed electrode is offered up to a block of metal and an electrical voltage applied. A spark jumps the gap and erodes the metal surface. This process can remove metal selectively with great accuracy. It is being applied in dentistry for the construction of crowns and bridges from titanium. A die is constructed of carbon and used as the electrode for the spark-erosion process. The outer surface of the crown is milled by a precision milling machine which traces the shape of a template to machine the shape into the titanium block.

Polishing

Polishing is usually accomplished by the abrasive action of rotary disks, brushes and pads, but some metal castings may be polished electrolytically. Cobalt chromium castings are often treated by this method. The casting is suspended in an electrolyte and a current passed through the system. At a microscopic level the 'tips of the mountains' of the rough surface are removed preferentially, leaving a smoother surface which is easier to fine polish afterwards.

Ultrasound cleaning

The principle of cavitation has already been described in the section on ultrasonic scalers. This effect is exploited once again in ultrasonic cleaning baths. Piezo electric crystal transducers are affixed to the base of a stainless steel bath filled with water. When the transducer is energised by a high-frequency alternating current, cavitation occurs in the water. Cavitation has a powerful cleaning effect on items placed into the tank.

Cleaning solutions of various types can be added to the tank to enhance the action of the ultrasound cleaning. The solution is specific to the material of construction of the items to be cleaned.

Ultrasonic cleaning baths are useful for cleaning up laboratory-made restorations prior to fitting at various stages in their construction. Ultrasonic baths are also used to disinfect dental impressions before they are cast up in the laboratory, to reduce the possibility of cross-infection. Special disinfecting solutions are used, the ultrasound ensuring full coverage and penetration of the solutions for maximum effectiveness.

Sandblasting

Metals can be cleaned readily by blasting the surface with an abrasive powder. Sandblasters propel abrasive grits through a nozzle at high velocity in a stream of compressed air. Sandblasters can be used to clean off residual investment materials and to prepare the metal surfaces for further treatments.

Sandblasting is usually carried out in a closed container fitted with a window and an interior light. Dust extraction systems keep the abrasive grit in the container and the most sophisticated can re-circulate it back through the blasting nozzle. Recirculation can degrade the grit rapidly and it can become much less effective. This has been shown to be of direct clinical relevence when metal surfaces are being roughened prior to bonding. The best and strongest bonds are formed when fresh grit is used.

Various grades of grit can be used. The finest grits will almost polish the surface of cast gold restorations and are very useful in finishing techniques.

Curing baths

Acrylic resin is used widely in dentistry, especially in the construction of dentures. The polymerisation of acrylic resin is achieved most effectively at elevated pressures and temperatures. Either or both of these conditions can be achieved by the use of various types of curing baths. The simplest curing bath for denture work is an electrically-heated water bath, the temperature of which is regulated by a thermostat. Elevated pressures can be achieved in small water-filled flasks which can be compressed in a bench-press to a high pressure. These are known as hydro-flasks.

High pressure and temperature water baths are also produced as self-contained units for use in post-curing composite materials for crown and inlay work. The concept is that under these conditions the level of conversion of monomer to polymer is greatly increased although the resultant improvement in the physical properties of the set material may be only slight.

Etching units

Metals can be bonded directly to teeth micro-mechanically by etching both the metal and the tooth to create a retentive pattern into which a bonding resin can run and set. The method of preparing the metal was developed at the University of Maryland, USA, and is known as etched metal and the clinical application is known as the Maryland Bridge.

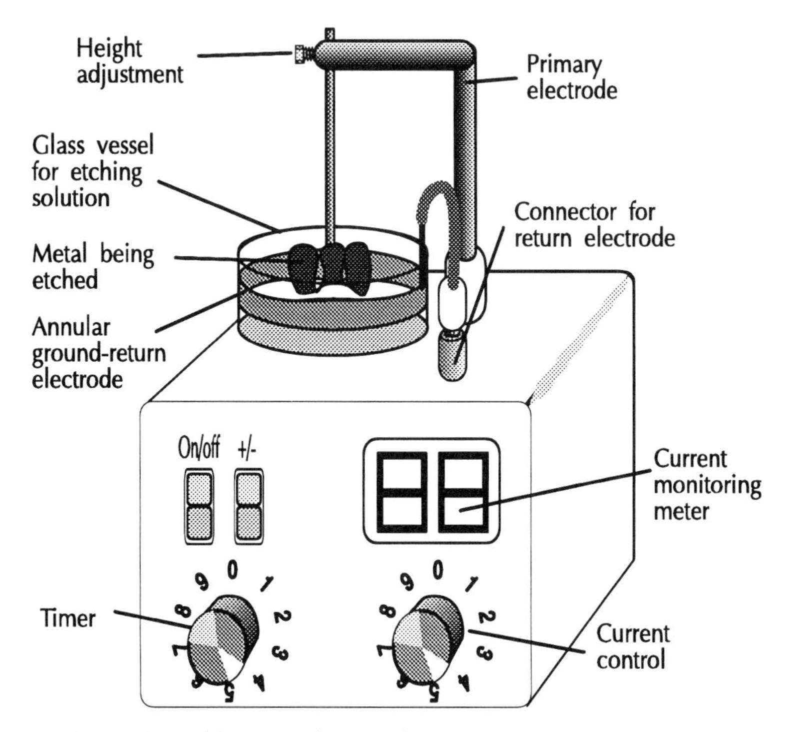

Fig. 118. Etching unit; layout of components.

When an alloy freezes after casting it forms in grains with grain boundaries. The metals constituent within the alloy are chosen so that those which are most chemically reactive concentrate within the grain boundaries. This makes the boundaries highly susceptible to corrosion in acid. By immersing the metal in an acid and passing an electrical current through it, the metal can be etched differentially. This differential etching creates deep pits within the metal surface into which the bonding resin flows.

The etching apparatus, illustrated in *Fig. 118,* consists of a current source with automatic timer and a system of connections for attaching the castings to be treated. Most etching units have automatic timers and some are programmed to reverse the current intermittently to clean the surface whilst the etching continues *(Fig. 119)*.

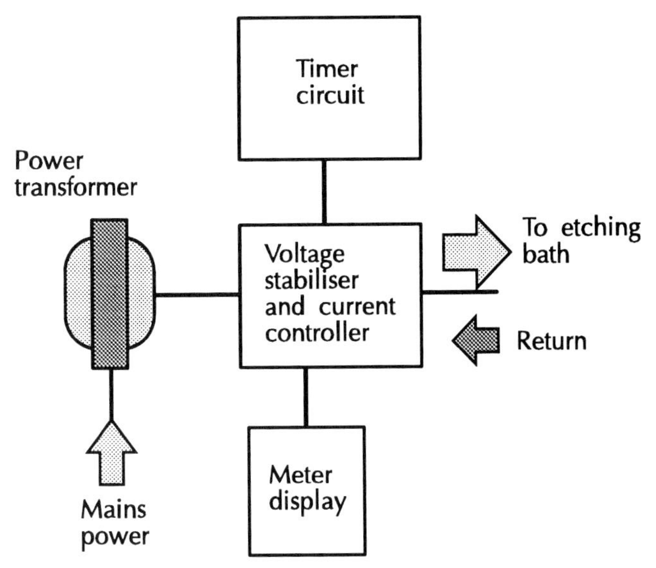

Fig. 119. Etching unit; electrical circuit.

Vacuum mixers

Plasters and stones are used for many purposes in the dental laboratory and it is often necessary to achieve a fine surface finish when casting models and investing dies. A fine surface can be achieved only if the plaster is free of air bubbles. This is especially important in investing patterns for casting because air bubbles in the investment lead to surface additions on the casting. The amount of air in a dental stone can be reduced by mixing the material under a partial vacuum. In this way any bubbles which are present will tend to explode at the surface of the material whilst it is being mixed. Any bubbles trapped in the material will shrink again after the material is exposed to atmospheric pressure before it has set.

A vacuum mixer consists of a mixing vessel which may be sealed hermetically and which contains a rotating mixing paddle. A vacuum pump is used to reduce the pressure in the vessel whilst a geared-down electric motor spins the paddle and mixes the material.

The most sophisticated mixers allow wax patterns to be invested under reduced pressure after the investment has been mixed.

Model-trimmers

Model-trimmers are devices used for cutting back the bases of plaster casts to a required shape. The device is based on a large rotating disk, usually at least 300 mm in diameter, which has a coarse abrasive surface and which turns at a high speed. A powerful electric motor is needed to turn the disk. The disk is enshrouded in a metal casing with a window onto its cutting surface. A platform at this window enables a plaster cast to be supported whilst it is trimmed *(Fig. 120)*.

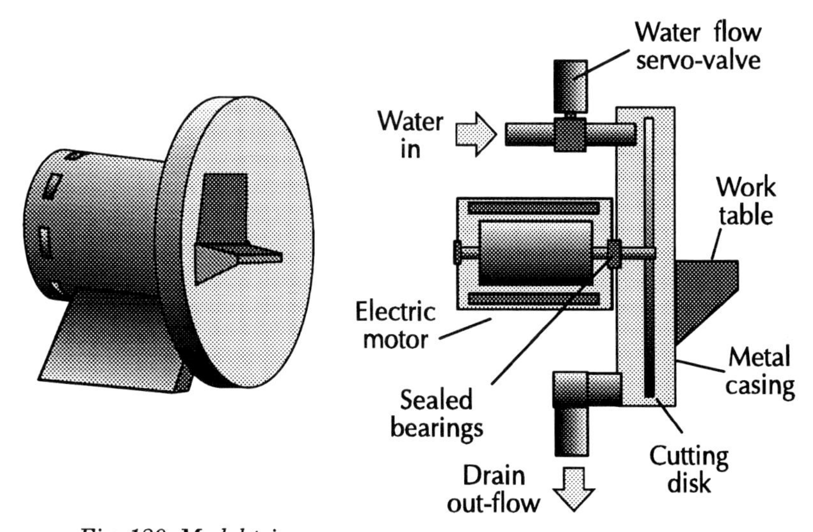

Fig. 120. Model trimmer.

Plaster would clog a disk up in a few revolutions if it wasn't removed and therefore water is flushed over the cutting disk whist it is in use to remove the debris. It is essential that care is taken to filter the drain water through a plaster-trap otherwise the out-flow can block up drains rapidly. Top quality machines use a servo-valve to switch the water supply at the same time as the motor. As with all servo-valves it is sensible to operate a manual tap to isolate the system when it is not in use or it is to be left unattended overnight. One such trimmer with a faulty servo-valve managed to flood several floors of our dental school when it failed early one weekend and was not discovered until the building was opened on Monday morning.

Vacuum-forming units

Vacuum-forming is used for the construction of splints, formers for temporary restorations, crown reduction guides, sports mouth-guards, bruxism splints, etc. Vacuum-forming is accomplished by heating a sheet of plastic until it flows and then applying either a vacuum below it or high pressure above it so that it is forced down onto a model which acts as a mould. Whilst it would be more appropriate to call the air-pressure system a 'pressure-forming unit', it is traditional to lump the whole technology together under the term vacuum-forming.

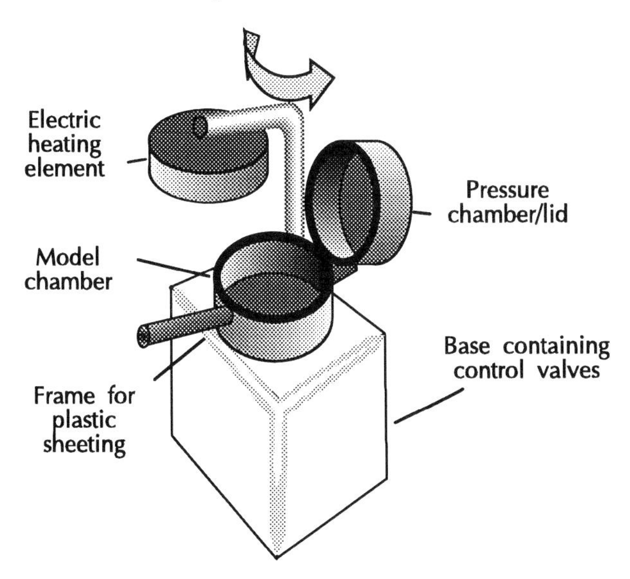

Fig. 121. Vacuum-forming unit.

Various plastics are used. Soft polyethylene is useful for formers for temporary restorations and for sports mouth-guards whilst harder and stiffer polycarbonate may be used for splinting purposes.

A typical unit is illustrated in *Fig. 121*. The model to be used as a mould is placed into a bed of lead shot within the pressure chamber. This allows the rapid displacement of air from the chamber whilst still supporting the model and the plastic sheeting. A plastic sheet of appropriate material is chosen and mounted in the frame over the model. An electrical heating element is swung into place and used to heat up and soften the plastic sheet. When the plastic begins to sag visibly, the heater is swung away and the top lid of the pressure chamber closed onto the plastic. The lid is pressurised with compressed air and forces the plastic sheet into tight contact with the model whereupon it cools. The lid is opened and the moulded sheet is removed from its frame and trimmed to shape.

CHAPTER 18

Basic Dental Research Technology

It is very difficult to cover the enormously wide range of experimental equipment used in dental research, but one or two items of equipment are in common use and are described in this section.

The optical microscope

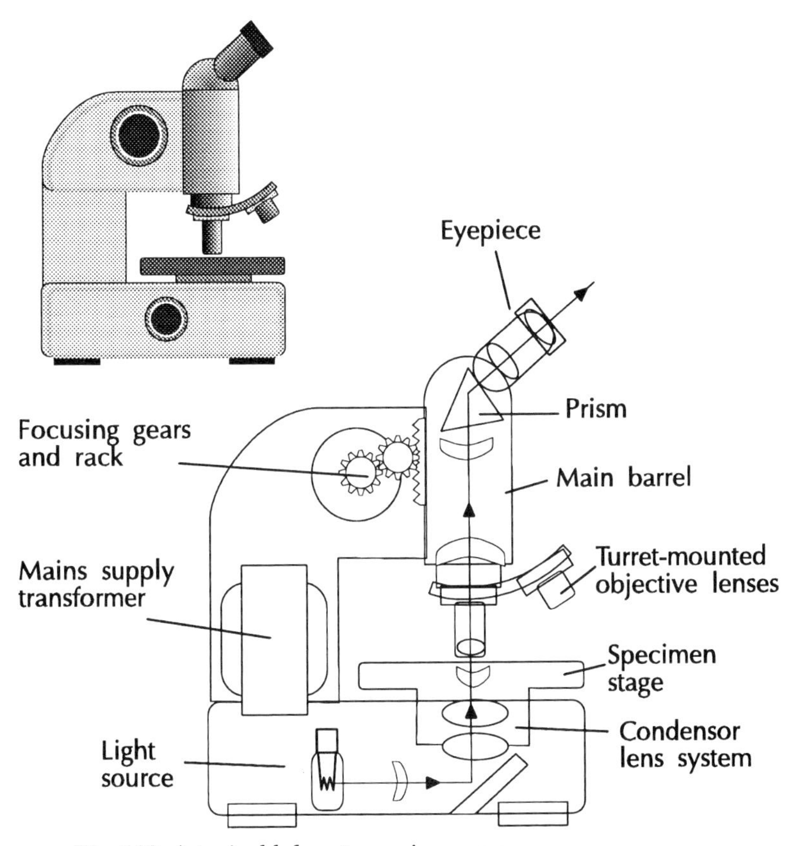

Fig. 122. A typical laboratory microscope.

The optical microscope remains a major research and teaching tool. An outline of a typical microscope is shown in *Fig. 122*. The magnification of a microscope is determined by the combination of objective lens and eyepiece, the two values being multiplied together to give the magnification of the combination. Most microscopes are capable of a range of magnification and this is usually accomplished by mounting a number of objective lenses of varying power on a rotating turret.

A further critical component is the light source. This is optimised to a clear even white background by a system of optics known as the condensor. This focuses the light from an incandescent bulb optimally for the particular objective lens in use.

Higher magnifications are obtained by eliminating the air gap between the objective lens and the specimen. A drop of oil is placed onto the specimen and then the microscope lens is lowered carefully into it. The oil has a refractive index radically different from air and enables clear focusing at high magnification. This is technique is known as oil-immersion.

Many specialised techniques have been developed for the examination of particular specimens. For example, polarised light reveals details of hard, crystalline materials. Certain specimens fluoresce under ultraviolet light and may require this form of illumination.

Optical microscopes are of little use above 2000 times magnification because the resolving power of light is limited by its wavelength. To go beyond this limit it is necessary to exploit shorter wavelengths of radiation and the electron microscope is used.

The electron microscope

The electron microscope is one of the fundamental devices for research. The light microscope is limited in resolution by the wavelength of light. In order to gain an increase in resolving power it is necessary to choose a radiation with a shorter wavelength. Electron beams provide the answer.

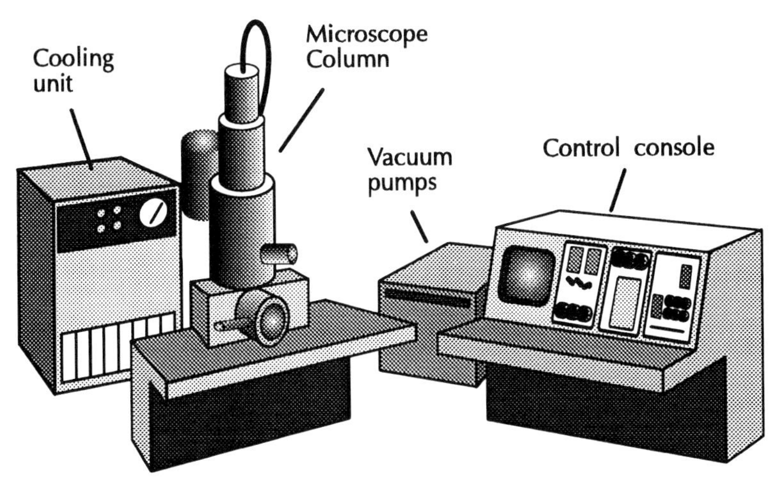

Fig. 123. A typical scanning electron microscope suite.

Electron microscopes operate in one of two ways, by transmission or by reflection.

Transmission electron microscopes operate by passing an electron beam through a very thin specimen and allowing it to create an image on a fluorescent screen or photographic film by direct projection.

Reflection electron microscopes cannot use a lens system for producing an image and require a different approach. The electron beam is focused into a very fine spot and then this spot is scanned across the specimen in a raster pattern. A detector detects the absorption or reflection of electrons at this point and a signal from this is fed to a television monitor. The raster of the TV image is matched to the raster of the electron beam scanning the specimen. In this manner an image of the specimen is created.

The main advantage of the scanning electron microscope *(Fig. 123)* is its ability to produce clear images with a tremendous depth of focus of solid objects.

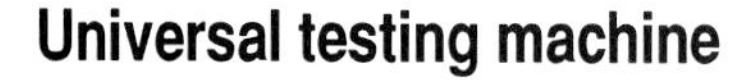

Universal testing machine

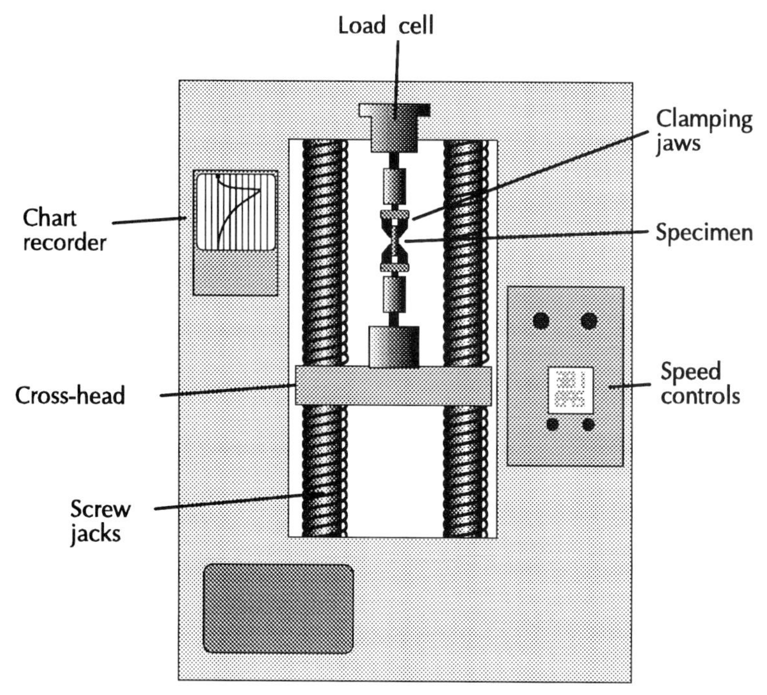

Fig. 124. Universal testing machine.

The universal testing machine *(Fig. 124),* often referred to by the trade name of the major manufacturer Instron, is an apparatus designed to test the mechanical properties of materials. The Instron subjects samples of materials or material systems to a load which is monitored continuously on a chart recorder. Effectively, the machine applies a strain to the test specimen and measures the stress. Tensile and compressive loads are applied by means of screw jacks which drive a cross-head within an overall supporting frame. The speed at which the cross-head moves is variable and is determined by a gear system and electronic control. Electronic load cells are interposed between the test specimen and the uppermost anchor point to monitor stress during compression or tension of the specimen. The most sophisticated models in the range are capable of applying torque loads as well. Loads can be increased continually to measure ultimate tensile strength and compressive strength. Intermittent loading can be cycled to measure fatigue effects.

Fatigue

The exposure of a material to a repetitive stress may lead to its failure at a value which reduces with time and the number of stress cycles. This is the effect of fatigue. Fatigue testing relates the amplitude of the stress to the number of cycles of stress needed to produce failure. The universal testing machine is often used to cycle loads in fatigue tests.

Rheometer

The viscosity of any material which can flow can be measured using a rheometer. One major application of the device in dentistry is to monitor the setting reactions of materials such as composites, polyalkanoates and impression materials. The most common form is the oscillating rheometer which applies an oscillating force to a test probe in the material to be measured. The resistance which the material offers to the oscillations of the rheometer can be used to calculate the viscosity. Other forms of rheometer trap a sample of material between contra-rotating disks and measure the drag to determine viscosity.

Hardness

Hardness is usually measured by means of an impact test. A diamond punch of known profile is delivered with a known force against the surface of the material to be tested. The deformation which is produced in the material is measured and this is used to give an index of hardness of the material.

Wear testing

Wear testing is an essential investigation on any new restorative material, but it is one of the most difficult tests to standardise. The wear of a surface will depend not only on the nature of the opposing wearing surface but also on any material interposed between. Many wear-tester devices have been developed but these rarely agree on a single standard. There have been many calls for standard methods to be established by the International

Standards Organisation so that wear testing can be compared across multiple independent evaluation.

Polarimetry and finite element analysis

Dental restorations are subjected to considerable loading and may fail for this reason. Similarly a tooth, damaged mechanically by cavity preparation, may fail structurally when loaded. Investigation of loading on a tooth is difficult in vivo so work is done mainly on simulation models.

Stress can be investigated in three ways; by strain gauges, photo-elastic models or by finite element analysis. Electrical or optical strain gauges can be applied to the surfaces of models and distortions measured. However this demonstrate stress at one point only and is therefore rather limited in usefulness.

Photo-elastic models and stress polarimetry are used in many areas of engineering science. A model of the structure to be investigated is made in a photo-elastic resin. These resins alter the polarisation of light shining through them when they are stressed. Light is passed through a polarising filter and then through the model. It is viewed through a polarising filter set at 90° to the illuminating filter. Light of different wavelengths rotates according to the levels of stress in the photo-elastic resin. Stress lines are revealed as coloured bands running across the model. By determining the colour shift the precise levels of stress in the model can be determined.

Finite element analysis is a method of stress analysis which uses a mathematical model of the structure. A sophisticated computer system is needed to create a useful model of dental structures. The system operates by dividing the model into a number of very small but discrete intersecting lines. This three-dimensional web has the overall shape of, for example, a tooth, but is built up of a number of very small lines. If properties such as the elastic modulus, the poisson ratio, etc. of the material is known, then the effect of applying a stress at one point can be calculated mathematically throughout the entire interlacing structure.

Creating an effective model is not without difficulty. Dental tissues have anisotropic properties, that is they are different depending on the orientation of the tissue. Furthermore, the boundaries between different structures, such as enamel and dentine, are very difficult to replicate. However, as computing power increases, more sophisticated and effective models can be created.

Index